KT-176-216

CLINICIAN'S GUIDE TO NUCLEAR MEDICINE

BRAIN BLOOD FLOW IN NEUROLOGY AND PSYCHIATRY

Clinician's Guide To Nuclear Medicine

Brain Blood Flow in Neurology and Psychiatry

D C Costa
Senior Clinical Lecturer and Honorary Consultant
Physician
The Institute of Nuclear Medicine
University College and Middlesex School of Medicine
London, UK

P J Ell
Head of Department
The Institute of Nuclear Medicine
University College and Middlesex School of Medicine
London, UK

CHURCHILL LIVINGSTONE
EDINBURGH • LONDON • MELBOURNE • NEW YORK 1991

CHURCHILL LIVINGSTONE
Medical Division of Longman Group UK Limited

Distributed in the United States of America by
Churchill Livingstone Inc., 1560 Broadway, New York,
N.Y. 10036, and by associated companies, branches
and representatives throughout the world.

© British Nuclear Medicine Society

All rights reserved; no part of this publication
may be reproduced, stored in a retrieval system,
or transmitted in any form or by any means,
electronic, mechanical, photocopying, recording
or otherwise, without either the prior written permission
of the Publishers (Churchill Livingstone, Robert Stevenson
House, 1–3 Baxter's Place, Leith Walk, Edinburgh EH1 3AF)
or a licence permitting restricted copying in the United Kingdom
issued by the Copyright Licensing Agency Ltd,
33–34 Alfred Place, London WC1E 7DP.

First published 1991

ISBN 0-443-04282-9

British Library Cataloguing in Publication Data available

Library of Congress Cataloging-in-Publication Data available

Produced by Longman Singapore Publishers Pte Ltd
Printed in Singapore

Preface

Nuclear medicine has an established place in modern medicine. The specialty is now almost 50 years old, the first clinically useful applications of the radioactive tracer method being developed in the late 1940s and early 1950s.

The scope of nuclear medicine has grown spectacularly in this period, but its nature has also altered due to the introduction and development of other imaging modalities, notably X-ray CT scanning, magnetic resonance imaging and diagnostic ultrasound. Nuclear medicine, however, remains unique in its ability to yield functionally rather than anatomically based, information.

This series of books entitled 'A Clinician's Guide to Nuclear Medicine' intends to present the clinical utility of Nuclear Medicine to all doctors, whether in general medicine/surgery or specialized disciplines.

Under the auspices of the British Nuclear Medicine Society, expert physicians from the United Kingdom have been asked to write these books. As the title of the series implies, the book should act as a guide to clinicians interested in the radioactive tracer method in their own specialty or in clinical practice. In general, a series Editor has co-ordinated this development, Amersham International plc has helped to sponsor the publication of these books, and Churchill Livingstone has been appointed as Publisher for this series.

The British Nuclear Medicine Society hopes that these books will help the clinician to understand the potential and wide-ranging applications of the radioactive tracer method to Medicine in general and to clinical problem-solving in particular.

The books are well illustrated, have been purposely designed as handbooks, and contain many useful tables and diagrams. The discussion of clinical case material is included, wherever relevant.

London, 1991   P J Ell

Acknowledgements

We wish to thank the following individuals and Institutions for their collaboration:

Institute of Neurological Sciences, Glasgow for their kind permission to include case studies 1 to 11.

Memory Clinic, Section of Old Age Psychiatry, Institute of Psychiatry and Professor Raymond Levy for referring patients with DAT and age matched controls.

Academic Unit of Neurosciences and Department of Nuclear Medicine, Charing Cross Hospital for the studies of patients with migraine.

Professor M G Harrison, Dr R Fish, Mr M Powell, Mr F Iannotti, Mr M S Choksey, Dr J D King and Dr Mary Robertson for referring patients whose brain studies are included.

The Department of Medical Photography (UCMSM), and Department of Medical Illustration (Charing Cross Hospital) for their help with some of the illustrations in this work.

The staff of the Institute of Nuclear Medicine, UCMSM for their help.

This series is sponsored by a Grant from Amersham International plc for which the authors, editor and the Council of the British Nuclear Medicine Society are thankful.

Contents

THE CLINICAL PROBLEM

Cerebrovascular disease is the third most common cause of death in the USA and Europe. The annual incidence of stroke rises with age, and it is greater than 1% per annum in those over 65 years old. However, in spite of an increasingly aging population and the prevalence and morbidity of cerebrovascular diseases as a whole, their natural history is rather poorly understood. Management is often subjective and based on clinical criteria alone, and little encouragement has been given to active forms of treatment, stroke care units, rehabilitation and controlled follow-up studies.

Between 3% and 5% of people over 65 suffer from impairment of memory, personality changes and mild dementia, the most common cause of which is Alzheimer's disease. While senile dementia is present in less than 1% of people under 65, it rises to more than 15% in those over 85. There is a clear age dependency of dementia and the prevalence of this disease is growing with the increased age of the population at large.

The study of cerebral blood flow is relevant to the clinical investigation of these and many other groups of patients. Examples of other patient groups in which blood flow assessment has proved useful include transient ischaemic attack (TIA), prolonged reversible ischaemia with neurological deficit (PRIND), focal epilepsy, trauma and migraine. In most circumstances, where new treatment regimes are being investigated for these groups of patients, cerebral blood flow studies could be expected to contribute to the monitoring of the patient status.

Measuring cerebral blood flow in man has led to an improved perception of the pathophysiology of cerebrovascular disease. In normal man, mean cerebral blood flow

(CBF) is kept constant by autoregulation, and varies between 50 and 60 ml/min/100 g of brain substance. The flow in normal grey matter is higher (65 to 85 ml/min/100 g) than in normal white matter (27 to 33 ml/min/100 g). Normal cerebral function is still possible with mean CBF values as low as 20 ml/min/100 g, the brain compensating with an increase in oxygen extraction from the circulation. Values below this limit lead to abnormalities detected by electroencephalography, but at 15 ml/min/100 g critical ischaemia is reached, and if prolonged, irreversible cellular damage will occur. During autoregulation, cerebral blood volume (CBV) can increase (through vessel dilation) at constant blood flow. When vessel dilatation is maximal and CBV can no longer increase, CBF begins to fall. It has been shown that combined studies of CBF and CBV record an index of cerebral perfusion reserve (Gibbs et al 1984) and clearly relate to the fractional oxygen extraction of the brain.

The assessment of cerebral blood flow would therefore appear to have an important role in both clinical research and routine patient management. However, the technique has never become widely established.

THE METHODOLOGICAL PROBLEM

While techniques for the measurement of cerebral blood flow in man have been available for many years, most of these have lacked spatial resolution and depth resolution. The ^{133}Xe planar method, in particular, on which most of the information on cerebral blood flow is based, has been shown to be insensitive and subject to artefacts, within the context of day-do-day clinical patient evaluation. Information display is in the form of maps of numbers (Ingvar & Lassen 1961) rather than images and information is only available for cerebral cortex with no data on deep brain structures. However, the great attraction of the planar ^{133}Xe CBF methodology remains its relative simplicity and even portability (Agnoli et al 1969, Rosenstein et al 1984).

At the opposite extreme of technical complexity, positron emission tomography (PET) is, at present, the most accurate technique designed to give regional quantitative information on brain perfusion and metabolism. The unique advantage of PET lies in its ability to provide a metabolic map of disease processes. Parameters such as oxygen extraction rate and glucose consumption can be measured, as well as blood flow. However, PET remains hugely expensive, generally unavailable on a routine basis for clinical investigation of patients, and at present, installed in a very limited number of centres.

The alternative approach to the regional and tomographic investigation of the brain in man lies with single photon emission computerized tomography (SPET). This technique can be carried out with conventional instrumentation or utilizing specially designed, dedicated equipment which is still a fraction of the cost of a multi-slice PET instrument.

SPET instrumentation has, over the recent past, improved significantly, with greater reliability, improved spatial resolution and contrast detail (some of this improvement will be noted in the pictorial section of this book). SPET is available in hundreds of centres in Europe and in many departments in the UK.

It is often stated that the difficulties encountered in quantification with SPET pose constraints to its wider utility. While in this volume, this issue will only be addressed in a rather limited fashion, it is of note that CBF/CBV studies are in progress with SPET and that the recorded results available from the literature resemble the results which have been obtained using PET technology (Knapp et al 1986). This is encouraging and this avenue of work will expand considerably in the near future. Ratios of count rate distributions may prove clinically useful, even when absolute values for CBF are more difficult to obtain.

However, the most important limitation to the widespread use of SPET in the clinical investigation of the neurological or psychiatric patient has been the lack of adequate and routinely available radiopharmaceuticals.

THE TRACER PROBLEM

The ideal radiopharmaceutical for the assessment of CBF must distribute according to flow, be widely available, lead to optimal utilization of the conventional rotating gamma camera, and permit repeat studies to be carried out, for which it must be both safe and inexpensive.

These aims have not been achieved in the past. Tomographic ^{133}Xe CBF studies require special purpose instrumentation, ^{123}I-labelled amines and diamines are costly and of limited availability and ^{201}Tl-diethyldithiocarbamate suffers from the poor physical and imaging properties of ^{201}Tl. This problem (and the first practical solution to it) has led to the recent development of a ^{99m}Tc-labelled tracer for the investigation of CBF in man.

REFERENCES

Agnoli A, Prencipe M, Priori AAM, Bozzao I, Fieschi C 1969 Measurements of rCBF by intravenous injection of 133-Xenon. In: Brock M, Fieschi C, Ingvar DH, Lassen NA, Schurmann K (eds) Cerebral Blood Flow, Springer-Verlag, Berlin, pp 31–34

Gibbs JM, Wise RJS, Leenders KL, Jones T 1984 Evaluation of cerebral perfusion reserve in patients with carotid artery occlusion. The Lancet **i:** 310–314

Ingvar DH, Lassen NA 1961 Quantitative determination of regional cerebral blood flow in man. The Lancet **ii:** 806–807

Knapp WH, Von Kummer R, Kubler W 1986 Imaging of Cerebral Blood Flow-to-Volume Distribution Using SPECT. Journal of Nuclear Medicine **27:** 465–470

Rosenstein J, Suzuki M, Symon L, Redmond S 1984 Clinical use of a portable bedside cerebral blood flow machine in the management of aneurysmal subarachnoid hemorrhage. Neurosurgery **15:** 519–525

DEVELOPMENT OF ^{99m}Tc-LABELLED TRACERS

Regional blood flow in an organ can be measured from the deposition, due to capillary blockade, of radioactively-labelled microspheres of an appropriate size (Marcus et al 1976). This technique has been used as a standard against which the capability of other techniques to assess regional cerebral blood flow (rCBF) has been compared (Wagner et al 1969, Warner et al 1987).

For routine clinical assessment of cerebrovascular diseases, capillary blockade is not a preferred option, and a 'chemical microsphere' is required as a compound which will be trapped in the brain without causing physical blockage. For the assessment of rCBF, this can be accomplished if the agent crosses the blood-brain barrier (BBB) and is retained in brain tissue. The distribution of a radiolabelled 'chemical microsphere' can be measured using readily available imaging equipment, in order to obtain a map of rCBF.

To cross the intact BBB, a molecule might employ one or a combination of three transport mechanisms:

1 Active transport
2 Facilitated transport by a carrier
3 Passive diffusion

Active transport and facilitated transport are highly structure-sensitive mechanisms, since they involve binding to carrier molecules. While it is possible to develop molecules labelled with positron emitting nuclides such as ^{11}C, ^{13}N, ^{15}O or even ^{18}F which can cross the BBB by these mechanisms and image rCBF, most practically useful isotopes are obtained from elements which normally do not occur in physiologically interesting molecules. This virtually eliminates the possibility that these molecules will be actively transported across the BBB. Therefore, labelled molecules suitable for routine rCBF imaging are restricted to those which may cross the BBB by passive diffusion.

The rate of passive diffusion depends on the size, charge and lipophilicity of a molecule. Small, hydrophobic molecules such as O_2, Xe and benzene, and small, uncharged, polar molecules such H_2O, CO_2 and glycerol cross the lipid bilayer readily. Ions such as H^+ or Na^+, and large uncharged polar molecules are virtually excluded. For example, the permeability of the cell membrane lipid bilayer for H_2O and K^+ differs by a factor of 10^{10}. However, it is not merely the membrane transport characteristics of a molecule which define its acceptability as an agent for assessment of rCBF.

A number of alternative imaging techniques are available for the assessment of the distribution of a gamma-emitting tracer. Tomographic imaging is preferred for an anatomically complex organ such as the brain, and the rotating gamma camera is the preferred instrument, as it is versatile, and more readily available. However a typical study with the rotating camera takes 20–30 minutes, during which time the distribution of radiolabelled tracer in the brain may vary only minimally.

The 'chemical microspheres' which cross the BBB have widely-varying clearance characteristics. Agents that remain unchanged within the brain, such as $H_2^{15}O$ and ^{133}Xe are cleared quickly, whereas other agents such as ^{123}I-iodo-amphetamine (^{123}IMP) and its related compounds, and ^{201}Tl-DDC (diethyldithiocarbamate) may be trapped in brain tissue. Until now, it is only this latter group which have proved useful for routine rCBF imaging.

Characteristics of the ideal agent

The ideal agent for the practical assessment of rCBF can be defined by the following characteristics:

1 The molecule should be neutral and lipophilic to enable passive diffusion across the lipid bilayer.
2 The extraction efficiency of the molecule must be high.
3 Once trapped, the distribution of the molecule must

remain effectively unchanged, at least over the time frame of the imaging procedure.

4 Clearance from brain tissue should be slow.

5 The radioisotope used should be continuously available and have physical characteristics suitable for high resolution gamma imaging.

6 The molecule must be easy to use and safe.

The ideal isotope is, of course ^{99m}Tc, the ubiquitous nuclide of nuclear medicine utilized in over 80% of all procedures. Much work has been carried out on molecules capable of transporting ^{99m}Tc across the intact BBB. However, very few molecules have been found which show this property. Most work has centred on the derivatives of propylene amine oxime (PAO), bisaminothiol (BAT) and kethoxal bisthiosemicarbazone (KTS) (Fig. 2.1).

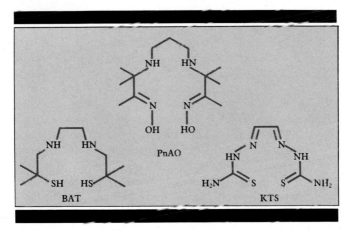

Fig. 2.1 **Ligands forming ^{99m}Tc complexes capable of crossing the BBB.**

All three of these ligands have been shown to form lipophilic Tc-complexes which are extracted into normal brain tissue (Fig. 2.2). However, they are not retained, and their distribution can only be measured using fast imaging ring devices such as the Medimatic Tomomatic range and the SME Tomograph. While these instruments can give excellent, high resolution tomographic images, they are

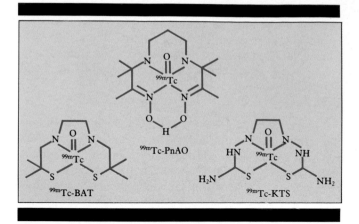

Fig. 2.2 **Neutral ^{99m}Tc complexes.**

expensive, dedicated and not yet widely available. The incorporation of a moiety to elicit trapping of the ^{99m}Tc complex is therefore required to give these molecules wide diagnostic utility.

Uptake
The permeability of lipid membranes depends not only on lipophilicity but also on the molecular weight of permeating molecules. Levin (1980) evaluated the capillary permeability coefficient, Pc, of a series of compounds and compared these with the theoretical values, calculated from the octanol/water partition coefficient, P, and the molecular weight (MW) of the compound. He found the following relationship:

$$\text{LogPc} = -4.605 + 0.4115 \log [P(MW)^{1.2}]$$

demonstrating the importance of both MW and lipophilicity as determinants of permeability through lipid membranes. He also determined a molecular weight cut-off for significant BBB passage as lying between 400 and 675 daltons.

Following the encouraging early work of the University of Missouri (Volkert 1984a,b), PAO was selected as a ligand having potential for further development. A series of PAO derivatives of increasing MW were subsequently synthesized (Fig. 2.3) whose in-vivo distribution studies confirmed Levin's findings (Table 2.1). However, in rats the relative brain uptake of these complexes fell very sharply between MW 468 and 524, despite an increase in lipophilicity. Over a limited MW range the effect on brain permeability could be negligible, and the sudden drop-off in brain intake of highly lipophilic molecules could reflect a very high affinity for blood proteins. As the measurements were carried out following i.v. injection this protein binding should be taken into account, and experiments have shown a dramatic increase in protein binding between $\log P = 0.5$ and $\log P = 3.5$. The sudden BBB permeability deterioration between $\log P = 4$ and $\log P = 6$ might reflect strong protein binding by such highly lipophilic molecules.

Trapping

To accomplish the trapping of a freely diffusible complex, either its lipophilicity must be altered as it enters the cell, or it must interact with an intracellular component such that diffusion back across the BBB is severely restricted. One approach to designing a molecule to be trapped in brain tissue is to attach to a known ligand a moiety which will interact with brain-selective mechanisms. For example, the trapping of amphetamine derivatives such as [123]IMP could be explained by interaction with specific brain

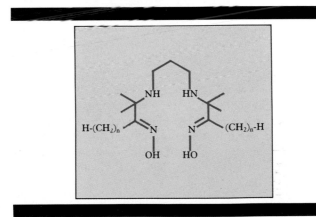

Fig. 2.3 **PAO derivatives of increasing molecular weight.**

Table 2.1 **Relationship between chain length, lipophilicity and brain uptake of PAO derivatives**

Chain length (n*)	Lipophilicity (Log P)	% Brain uptake in rats
1	1.0	0.92±0.05
2	2.0	0.85±0.02
3	2.7	0.72±0.13
4	3.1	1.22±0.12
5	–	0.23±0.03
6	5.6	0.11±0.0
8	6.8	0.12±0.0
9	7.2	0.20±0.03

* See Fig. 2.3

receptors, with monoamine oxidases, or with low selectivity, high capacity proteins inside the brain (Winchell et al 1980). Alternatively the trapping of the selenium-containing PIPSE and MOSE has been explained in terms of the 'pH shift' phenomenon (Kung et al 1980) in which a change of lipophilicity takes place within the brain due to the higher acidity (lower pH) compared with blood.

A series of amine derivatives of PAO were synthesized (Fig. 2.4), the ^{99m}Tc-complexes of which had the appropriate pKa to allow trapping according to the pH shift theory; results, however, show a lack of brain uptake and retention (Table 2.2). PAO derivatives (which are substrates for monoamine oxidases), esters (which are substrates for esterases), and dihydropyridine derivatives (which are sensitive to intracerebral oxidation) were also evaluated but the results were disappointing. The lack of brain uptake of these compounds, even at 2 minutes post-injection, is probably due to the addition of heteroatoms onto the PAO core. According to Partridge (personal communication) log P(MW), which controls the membrane permeability of a compound, decreases when the number of hydrogen bonds which the compound forms in aqueous solution increases; heteroatoms added to the PAO core will therefore decrease the permeability.

THE DEMETHYLATED PAO SERIES

A breakthrough came with the synthesis at Amersham

Table 2.2 **Substituted PAO derivatives and brain uptake in rats**

Substituents			% Brain uptake
R_3	R_4	R_1, R_7	
N-piperidinyl	H	Me	0.12±0.04
N-piperidinyl	H	n-Bu	0.27±0.03
N-morpholinyl	H	Me	0.17±0.02
N-morpholinyl	H	Et	0.14±0.0
2-N-morpholinylethyl	H	Me	0.20±0.03
2-N-ethylanilinoethyl	H	Me	0.03±0.1
2-pyridyl	H	Me	0.1±0.06
aminomethylene	Me	Me	0.06±0.03
aminomethylene	Me	n-Bu	0.06±0.02
N-isopropylamino methylene	Me	Me	0.07±0.02

$R_1 = R_2 = R_5 = R_6 = $ Me.

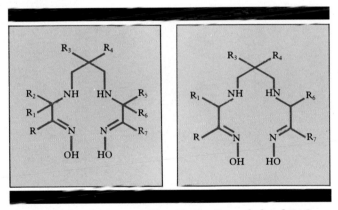

Fig. 2.4 **Amine derivatives of PAO.**

Fig. 2.5 **Demethylated PAO series.**

International of a series of PAO-type ligands which had relatively unstable Tc-complexes (Fig. 2.5). These ligands have the common feature that $R_2 = R_5 = $ H on the PAO ligand (Fig. 2.4) while R, R_1, R_6 and R_7 are alkyl groups. Chemical instability can be found in all ^{99m}Tc-complexes of PAO-type ligands but is especially marked with the demethylated compounds, such that conversion to less lipophilic species occurs even in aqueous medium containing only the complex, excess ligand and a small amount of stannous chloride. The conversion rate can be greatly accelerated by the addition of reducing agents.

HMPAO

The structures of the most interesting demethylated PAO derivatives are shown in Table 2.3. Preliminary extraction efficiency data suggested that the ^{99m}Tc-complex of HMPAO would be the superior molecule, and its biodistribution in rats indicated it to be well retained in brain tissue. An inspection of the HMPAO molecule reveals the existence of *meso* and *d,l* diastereoisomers (Fig. 2.6) and the in-vivo distribution in rats of ^{99m}Tc-labelled complexes of the separated isomers indicated the superiority of the *d,l* form over the *meso* isomer for imaging with the rotating gamma camera (Table 2.4).

Table 2.3

R_1, R_7	R_1, R_6	R_3, R_4	PAO-derivative
Me	Me	H	TM-PAO
Me	Me	Me	HM-PAO
Me	Et	H	DMDE-PAO
Et	Me	Me	DETM-PAO
Me	Me	Et	TMDE-PAO

Table 2.4 **Biodistribution of HMPAO isomers in the rat**

% dose	Time post-injection (mins)							
	d,l-isomer				*meso*-isomer			
	2	10	30	60	2	10	30	60
Brain	2.1	2.1	1.8	2.0	1.1	0.7	0.7	0.6
Blood	11.0	10.0	9.3	8.7	5.0	3.8	3.4	2.7
Muscle	23.6	32.6	23.4	17.4	29.2	18.9	13.6	10.9
Liver+GI tract	29.3	26.0	30.2	30.2	39.6	51.0	61.1	62.4
Kidneys+urine	7.6	9.5	16.4	21.0	3.2	3.2	5.8	9.9

Values are the mean of 2 or 3 rats at each time point

In-vitro data revealed the greater instability of ^{99m}Tc-*d,l*-HMPAO [conversion rate in aqueous medium Rc = 2.2 × 10^{-3} min^{-1}] compared with ^{99m}Tc-*meso*-HMPAO [Rc = 10^{-3}

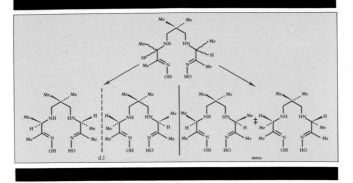

Fig. 2.6 **Meso** and **d,l** diastereoisomers of HMPAO.

min⁻¹] and PAO [Rc = 10⁻⁴ min⁻¹]. First clinical studies at the Middlesex Hospital Medical School (Ell et al 1985a,b) with a mixture of isomers, subsequently extended by the University of Aberdeen (Sharp et al 1986) using the separated isomers (Fig. 2.7), confirmed that ⁹⁹ᵐTc-HMPAO and in particular the *d,l* isomer, was well retained in human brain with clearance of less than 1% per hour (Fig. 2.8). As a result of such studies, ⁹⁹ᵐTc-*d,l*-HMPAO had been demonstrated to be the current agent of choice for routine assessment of rCBF.

***Ceretec*ᵀᴹ** A technetium 'cold' kit has been formulated to provide an injectable solution of ⁹⁹ᵐTc-*d,l*-HMPAO following reconstitution with sterile ⁹⁹ᵐTc generator eluate. Ceretec is a lyophilized formulation containing 0.5 mg *d,l*-HMPAO, 7.6 μg stannous chloride dihydrate and 4.5 mg sodium chloride sealed in a glass vial under a nitrogen atmosphere. Each vial can be reconstituted with 5 ml of fresh ⁹⁹ᵐTc generator eluate containing up to 1.11 GBq (30 mCi) of ⁹⁹ᵐTc. Quality control tests for radiochemical purity (RCP), performed using thin-layer chromatography have shown a mean lipophilic complex content of ⁹⁹ᵐTc-*d,l*-HMPAO of 88±5% immediately following reconstitution. At 30 minutes post-reconstitution the value remains above 80%.

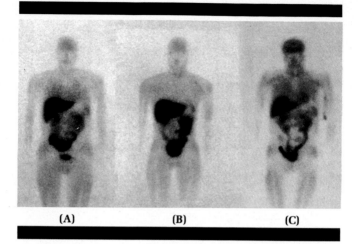

(A)   (B)   (C)

Fig. 2.7 **(A) Anterior view whole-body scan of** [99mTc]**-HMPAO mixture taken 4 hr post-injection. Uptake is seen in brain, skeletal muscle, and lung. Excretion is hepatobiliary; kidneys, bladder, liver, and small intestine are all visible. (B) Anterior view whole-body scan of** *meso* **isomer 4 hr post-injection. Distribution of material is similar to mixture but with lower lung uptake and obvious concentration of material in lachrymal glands. Brain uptake is only slightly higher than in soft tissue. (C) Anterior view whole-body scan of** *d,l* **isomer 4 hr post-injection. High brain uptake is clearly seen, as is uptake in myocardium, skeletal muscle of buttocks and medial aspect of thighs. Retention of material in left brachiocephalic vein is also apparent. Some trapping of material in the vein into which material is injected is a common feature of these materials. There is large urinary bladder activity and some retention in intestine.**

Human in vivo biodistribution

The human distribution pattern (Costa et al 1986, Sharp et al 1986) reflects the findings in rats. In man, approximately 5–6% of the injected dose localizes in the brain, and about 86% of this activity remains 24 hours after injection. The kidneys excrete 41% of the injected dose over the first 48 hours, and between 8.5 and 13.0% passes through the liver, enabling the main bile ducts and gall bladder to be

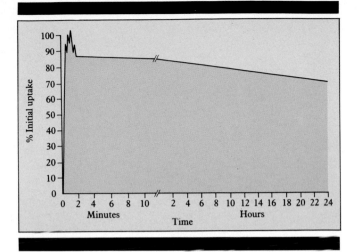

Fig. 2.8 **Retention of ^{99m}Tc-*d,l*-HMPAO in human brain over 24 hours (Tyrrell 1985).**

visualized. Lung uptake averages 9%, and about 2% of activity was seen in the myocardium of volunteers.

Dosimetry

Table 2.5 lists the organ dose estimates for the various body organs of a 70 kg adult following i.v. administration of ^{99m}Tc-HMPAO, in terms of mGy per 500 MBq dose (Soundy et al 1985). The organs receiving maximum dose are the lachrymal glands (35 mGy), gall bladder wall (27 mGy), kidneys (19 mGy), thyroid (15 mGy), and upper large intestine wall (14 mGy). The brain receives approximately 4 mGy and whole body dose is approximately 2 mGy. In all of these cases pessimistic assumptions were made regarding the activity distribution for modelling purposes.

Toxicology

Early clinical studies confirmed the biological behaviour of ^{99m}Tc-HMPAO in man to be very similar to that in the rat. Thus urinary excretion at 24 and 48 hours was virtually identical, and the general distribution throughout the body

Table 2.5

Target organ	Absorbed radiation dose (mGy per 500MBq)
Lachrymal glands	34.7
Gall bladder wall	27.3
Kidney	18.5
Thyroid	15.0
Upper large intestine wall	13.7
Liver	8.9
Small intestine wall	7.8
Lower large intestine wall	5.9
Urinary bladder wall	5.4
Brain	3.8
Ovaries	3.2
Testes	0.6
Whole body	2.1

was qualitatively similar. Allowing for the fact that many kinetic processes are faster in smaller animals, the quantitative distribution in rats at 1 hour approximated reasonably to that in humans between 2 and 8 hours, and the graph of blood clearance shows a very close agreement between normal human volunteers and male rats. The principal differences between the pharmacokinetic behaviour of ^{99m}Tc-HMPAO in rats and man is in the rate (and possible extent) of faecal elimination, and in the percentage of the dose taken up by the brain. The difference in brain uptake is presumably a reflection of the larger percentage of cardiac output which is delivered to the human brain.

Qualitative studies using a gamma camera confirmed that ^{99m}Tc-HMPAO crosses the rabbit blood-brain barrier and is retained in brain tissue, as in rat and man.

The intravenous route of administration was selected for toxicity studies since this represents the route of clinical exposure and guarantees complete systemic delivery of the test compound.

Acute toxicity Groups of male and female rats received either 1200 × maximum human dose (MHD), 100 × MHD or control vehicle. At necropsy there were no visible abnormalities and, quantitatively, no significant differences between the weights of brain, liver or kidneys from any of the dosage groups.

A similar study in rabbits produced similar results. No reactions to treatment were observed at the high (1200 × MHD) or low (100 × MHD) dose levels.

Chronic (repeat dose) toxicity In repeat dose studies, groups of male and female rats and rabbits received 14 consecutive daily injections of ^{99m}Tc-HMPAO. The total dose received by the highest dose group was equivalent to the administration of 14000 vials to a 70 kg human.

The results showed no treatment-related effects on weight gain, and no ophthalmologic effects. The blood chemistry values measured were within the normal range for the species; urinalysis in both rat and rabbit was largely unaffected. Necropsy showed the absence of histopatho-logical abnormalities in the brain and pituitary of rats and rabbits.

In conclusion, acute and repeat dose studies showed that, at the dosage levels studied, no treatment-related effects were elicited.

REFERENCES

Costa DC, Ell PJ, Cullum ID, Jarritt PH 1986 The *in vivo* distribution of ^{99m}Tc-HMPAO in normal man. Nuclear Medicine Communications 7: 647–658

Ell PJ, Cullum ID, Costa DC, et al 1985a A new regional cerebral blood flow mapping with ^{99m}Tc-labelled compound. The Lancet **ii**: 50–51

Ell PJ, Hocknell JML, Jarritt PH, et al 1985b A ^{99m}Tc-labelled radiotracer for the investigation of cerebral vascular disease. Nuclear Medicine Communications **6**: 437–441

Kung HF, Blau M 1980 Regional intracellular pH shift: a proposed new mechanism for radiopharmaceutical uptake in brain and other tissues. Journal of Nuclear Medicine **21**: 147–152

Levin VA 1980 Relationship of octanol/water partition coefficient and molecular weight to rat brain capillary permeability. Journal of Medicinal Chemistry **23**: 682–684

Marcus ML, Heistad DD, Ehrhardt JC, Abboud FM 1976 Total and regional cerebral blood flow measurement with 7-10-, 15-, 25-, and 50-μm microspheres. Journal of Applied Physiology **40:** 501–507

Sharp PF, Smith FW, Gemmell HG, et al 1986 Technetium-99m HMPAO stereoisomers as potential agents for imaging regional cerebral blood flow: human volunteer studies. Journal of Nuclear Medicine **27:** 171–177

Soundy RG, Tyrrel DA, Pickett RD 1985 Radiation doses to patients following intravenous injection with Technetium-99m-HMPAO. Amersham Report PTN 85/8, Corporate Safety Group Technical Note, (Internal Dose Calculation n.34)

Tyrrell DA 1985 Amersham Report N109/28. European Phase I and Phase II Clinical Trials.

Volkert WA, Hoffman TJ, Seger RM, Troutner DE, Holmes RA 1984a ^{99m}Tc-propylene amine oxime (^{99m}Tc-PnAO); a potential brain radiopharmaceutical. European Journal of Nuclear Medicine **9:** 511–516

Volkert WA, McKenzie EH, Hoffman TJ, Troutner DE, Holmes RA 1984b The behaviour of neutral amine oxime chelates labelled with Tc at tracer level. International Journal of Nuclear Medicine and Biology **11:** 243–246

Wagner HN Jr. Rhodes BA, Sasaki Y, Ryan JP 1969 Studies of the circulation with radioactive microspheres. Investigative Radiology **4:** 374–384

Warner DS, Kassell NF, Boarini DJ 1987 Microsphere cerebral blood flow determination. In: Wood JH (ed) Cerebral Blood Flow – Physiological and Clinical Aspects, McGraw-Hill, New York, pp. 288–298

Winchell HS, Horst WD, Braun L, Oldendorf WH, Hattner R, Parker H 1980 N-Isopropyl [^{123}I]-p-Iodoamphetamine: single-pass brain uptake and washout; binding to brain synaptosomes; and localization in dog and monkey brain. Journal of Nuclear Medicine **21:** 947–952

3 | SPET Measurements

In conventional radionuclide imaging the data is purely two-dimensional with no information obtained about the depth of sources within the object. In an attempt to reduce this problem, data is often taken from different positions around the object and the series of images (ie anterior, posterior, left and right laterals) then viewed as a set. As more views are taken so, at least in theory, should the localization of objects be improved. However, this is offset, first by the time which would be required to obtain the data and second, by the ever increasing number of images to be viewed. The other problem with conventional imaging is that each view represents the sum of activity (modified by attenuation) at all depths in the source, leading to a reduction of contrast in the image which is more severe the smaller the object (Fig. 3.1).

SPET

Single photon emission computerized tomography (SPET) is a natural extension of the multi-view technique described above. Data is acquired at a number of equally-spaced orientations around the patient (views or projections), but rather than look at each image separately, all the data is combined and 'reconstructed' to form images representing a plane in the patient. The time taken for each image is far less than for a conventional scan and hence the image quality of an individual projection is poor. The normal orientation of the reconstructed plane is transverse, but data in any plane, both perpendicular or oblique to the transverse, can be obtained (Fig. 3.2).

There are three theoretical advantages of SPET over planar scintigraphy, of which the first two below, have been realised.

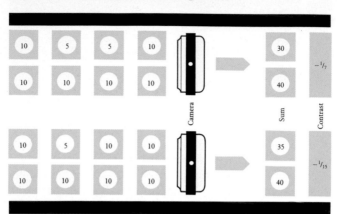

Fig. 3.1 **Reduction of image contrast due to overlying/underlying tissues.**

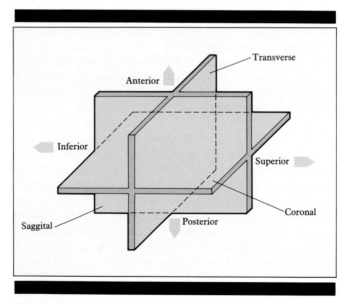

Fig. 3.2 **Principal image reconstruction planes.**

1 The positional information is truly three-dimensional, although it is normally viewed as a series of two-dimensional slices, each at a different position in the third dimension. This allows accurate length and volume

measurements (Kan & Hopkins 1979, Kuhl et al, 1980, Shapiro et al 1980) to be made over a wide range of object sizes, limited only at the low end by system resolution. Clinically, the superior positional information also allows better localization of lesions (for example whether in skull or brain) than when using planar scintigraphy alone.

2 Due to the effect of overlying and underlying tissues being largely (although not completely) eliminated, the contrast in SPET images is much higher than in equivalent planar views.

3 Radioisotope techniques trace a physiological pathway which is often related not only to the spatial distribution of the tracer but also to its absolute uptake. SPET should offer the ability, which planar scintigraphy does not, to quantify easily the activity of tracer within any part of any object. At present this potential has only been realized in a few, specialized, situations where the machine still requires calibration with a realistic phantom (Macey & Marshall 1982, Ell et al 1980).

HOW IS SPET PERFORMED?

The basic requirement for the formation of SPET images is the collection of data from a number of different angles (projections) around the object. The number of projections required depends on the information contained in any one projection and the desired image quality. However, a major distinction can be made between machines which collect data over an arc of at least 180 degrees (Full Angle Tomography) and those which employ a smaller angular range (Limited Angle Tomography). The full angle machines have been further sub-divided using various criteria, ie single or multi-dimensional instruments, special or general purpose instruments, multi- or single slice instruments where the positional data is obtained purely from the physical position of the detector and those where the detector itself supplies positional information, etc.

Following data acquisition, the projections are combined to produce a series of tomographic images ('slices'). This process is termed 'image reconstruction' and a very brief description of the main methods is given in a later section.

The instruments which are presently available to perform SPECT are outlined below.

Limited angle systems

These systems consist purely of special collimators which are attached to a standard Anger gamma camera and can be supplied by most collimator manufacturers. Image reconstruction algorithms are normally supplied by the user. The systems use the technique employed in conventional X-ray tomography, namely that objects at the same lateral location, but at different distances away from the camera, appear shifted with respect to each other when viewed from different angles (Fig. 3.3). The main attraction of the limited angle systems is that they are inexpensive and can be used with a standard gamma camera retaining its conventional imaging capability.

These systems are sometimes referred to as longitudinal tomographic devices, as their imaging plane is parallel to the face of the camera, rather than perpendicular to it as in full angle (transverse) systems. There have been two major collimator designs aimed at producing these different views of the object.

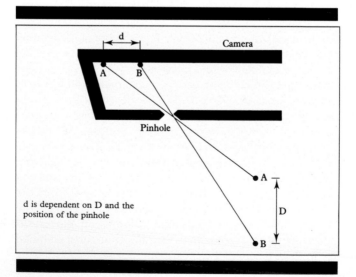

Fig. 3.3 **The basis of longitudinal tomographic systems.**

Seven pinhole collimator This collimator is used to split the camera face into seven sections, each of which views the object through a pinhole, providing seven views from slightly different angles (Fig. 3.4). No movement of the device is required to obtain all the data necessary to produce tomographic slices. The field of view of the system is limited to a volume where all the pinholes can 'see' the object. This consists of a cone-shaped region (Fig. 3.5) which causes difficulty in positioning objects and limits the size of objects which may be imaged.

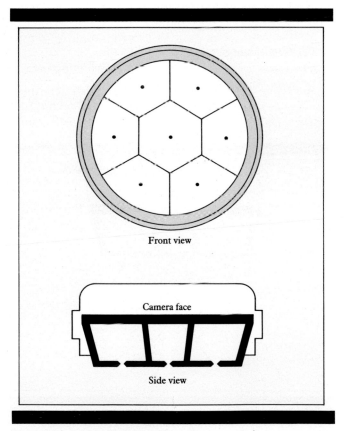

Front view

Camera face

Side view

Fig. 3.4 **The seven pinhole collimator.**

Rotating slant hole collimator This collimator consists of parallel holes which are slanted with respect to the face of the gamma camera (Fig. 3.6), data from different angles being acquired by rotating the collimator on the face of the camera after each view is obtained. Any number of such views may be obtained, with normally four views (each separated by 90 degrees) acquired.

Full angle systems

Rotating gamma cameras The key features of this system are as follows:

1 Single (or not many) detectors
2 Normally general purpose
3 Multi-slice
4 Positional data obtained from detector
5 Often useful for both brain and body scanning

Produced by most gamma camera manufacturers, these devices use a standard Anger gamma camera mounted on a special gantry which allows the camera to rotate around

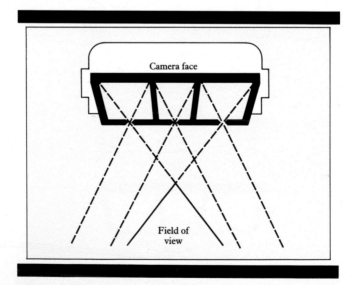

Fig. 3.5 **Cross section through the field of view of a seven pinhole collimator.**

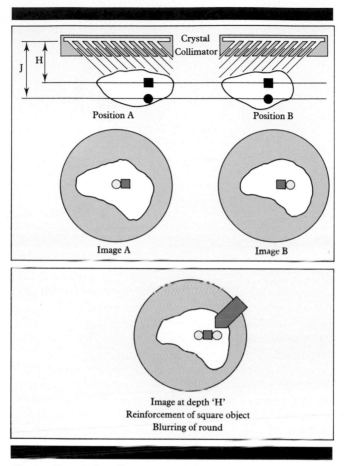

Fig. 3.6 **Slant hole collimator system.**

the object (Fig. 3.7). A series of images is obtained at equal angular spacing around the object, either by continuous rotation (slightly blurring out the data over a small angular range), or by stopping the camera at equal increments, obtaining data, and then moving on to the next position (the so called 'step and shoot' mode which misses data from the angles between each view). To reconstruct images, data is acquired from 180 degrees around the patient although, to minimize the effects of attenuation, 360-degree

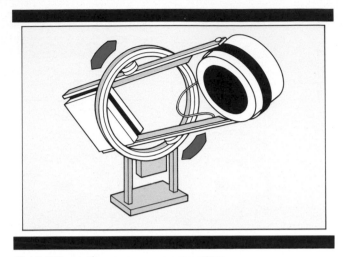

Fig. 3.7 **A rotating gamma camera system.**

rotation is normally used and opposing views combined to form a projection at that angle. In cases of small objects located near the surface of the body (for example the heart), 180-degree rotation, centred about the object, is often employed.

As with any gamma camera acquisition, image quality is improved by reducing the distance between the detector and the object. The standard, circular, orbit of the camera is not ideal in this respect, as the diameter of the circle is defined by the longest dimension of the object. An improvement in image quality can be obtained by performing 'elliptical orbits' which involve moving the camera (or the object) along a line perpendicular to the camera face so that the object is as near to the face of the camera as possible at all times. In the case of head scanning, it is normally the patient's shoulders which prevent the camera from moving close to the patient's head though there are two solutions to this problem. One is to use a 'cut-off' gamma camera head which is shortened so as not to reach the shoulders. The alternative is to use a slant hole collimator which allows the camera head to be tipped away from the shoulders (the direction of the holes defining the imaging plane) (Fig. 3.8).

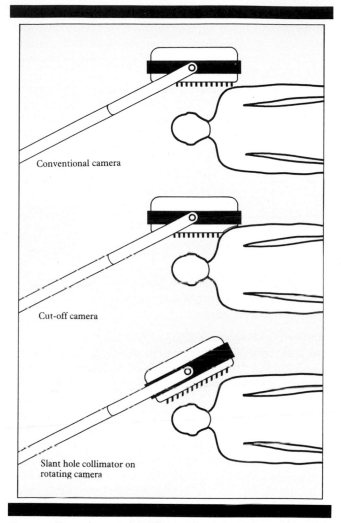

Fig. 3.8 **Alternative approaches to head scanning.**

To improve the sensitivity of the system (and hence reduce the scanning time required to produce an image of a given quality), the number of camera heads can be increased. Systems have employed two heads (Siemens), and three heads (TRIAD, NEUROCAM) while four would appear the logical maximum. However, due to the physical size of each detector, the three- and four-head systems may not be able to move as near to the object as is desirable (especially for head scanning). System parameters can also be varied to some extent by changing the collimator which is attached to the camera.

To remain a general purpose instrument the camera system must retain its ability to perform conventional imaging. This can be compromized by the design of the rotary gantry or by the time required to perform adjustments to the alignment of the system after it has been used conventionally (this is particularly important for multi-head systems).

SME 810 brain scanner The key features of this system are as follows:

1 Multi-detector
2 Special purpose
3 Single slice
4 No positional information from detector
5 Brain scanning only

Produced by Strichman Medical Equipment, this scanner is unique (with the exception of its direct predecessors, the Cleons 710 and 711) in that each detector yields information about the depth of sources via the use of short-focused collimators. There are twelve sodium iodide detectors in the system (in six opposed pairs), each fitted with two photomultiplier tubes providing energy, but no positional information. Each detector performs a rectilinear scan such that the focal point of the collimator passes across the whole object and through approximately half its depth, a projection being formed by the combination of the data from opposed detectors. The total number of projections from such a scan is six, but the angular sampling may be improved to twelve or eighteen projections by repeating the scanning procedure with the whole gantry rotated through the appropriate angle. To obtain information from different levels in the object, at the end of a scanning sequence the object is moved through the gantry by a set amount and the process repeated. The collimators are focused in both directions, in the data acquisition plane to obtain the depth information and perpendicular to it to increase sensitivity within the single slice being scanned.

The characteristics of this system can be altered by changing the collimators, allowing a trade-off between system resolution and sensitivity in an attempt to produce the best results in any clinical situation.

Tomomatic 32/64   The key features of this system are as follows:
1   Multi-detector
2   Special purpose
3   Single/multi-slice
4   No limited positional information from detector
5   Brain scanning only

These two systems, produced by Medimatic (Denmark) consist of four banks of sodium iodide detectors arranged in a square. To improve linear sampling, each bank of detectors is offset from its neighbours by one quarter of the detector spacing. In the 32-detector system, each detector is fitted with a single collimator focused at the centre of the object, while the 64-detector system has either three or five such collimators, enabling data to be obtained from three or five 'slices' simultaneously (Fig. 3.9). To enable the Tomomatic 64 to obtain this multi-slice data, one-dimensional positioning information is obtained from a set of photomultiplier tubes viewing the crystal. In operation the gantry rotates at high speed, collecting projection data as it does so. Images are generally reconstructed from the average of five or six such rotations.

As with the SME, 'slices' at different positions in the object are obtained by moving it with respect to the gantry at the end of the scanning sequence. The machine's characteristics may be altered by changing the collimation system employed.

Image reconstruction
In nearly all cases image reconstruction is performed by computer, although other techniques, eg optical, can be employed in certain circumstances.

Longitudinal systems   Here, the reconstruction algorithm

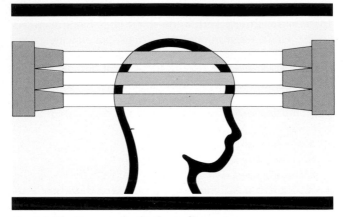

Fig. 3.9 **The Tomomatic 64, three slice system.**

has to apply a linear shift to each image and then sum this shifted dataset. The size of the shift applied determines the plane where data from each image is reinforced, other planes being blurred out. The effect of the blurred planes can, at least partially, be removed by a subsequent background subtraction. More sophisticated algorithms attempt to perform the reconstruction more precisely, but generally the contribution from other planes is never fully eliminated and hence the techniques cannot accurately quantify the activity in an object.

Full angle systems Here, two types of reconstruction technique are employed. The first type (analytical) involves mathematical manipulation of the project data followed by their superposition. The second type (iterative) involves successive approximations to the true image, each approximation being modified by comparing the projections it would produce with the true data.

The main advantage of the analytical methods is that they are fairly easily implemented and require only limited computing power, whereas the iterative techniques are more cumbersome and time-consuming. However, with recent improvements in computer hardware, iterative techniques are now a feasible option and their ability to incorporate system response functions and attenuation maps is likely to see them become the method of choice in the near future. (For detailed descriptions of the techniques, see Bracewell & Riddle 1967, Brooks & Di Chiro 1976, Budinger & Gullberg 1974, Cormack 1973, Gordon et al 1970, Herman & Rowland 1971, Kay et al 1974, Kemp 1980, Keyes et al 1973, Shepp & Logan 1974).

SYSTEM PERFORMANCE PARAMETERS

Many different methods have been used to assess machine performance, some of which, although giving a benchmark to compare different machines, have very little practical importance. In particular, the measurements of resolution performed with high contrast sources may bear very little relationship to the apparent resolution in clinical images, and high sensitivity values can result from wide energy windows or poor energy resolution. A brief description of the main performance characteristics is given below.

Resolution

One standard method of measurement is by the Full Width at Half Maximum (FWHM) or the Full Width at Tenth Maximum (FWTM) of the image of a thin line source perpendicular to the imaging plane (Fig. 3.10). This measurement can be misleading as, in a back projection reconstruction, very high resolution filters can be used while an iterative reconstruction can obtain a perfect imaging (one pixel resolution) due to low noise and no interfering structures. It is important to measure the resolution at different positions in the field of view and also at different orientations through the reconstructed image (for example the image of a circular source may not be round). The value measured will alter in the presence of a scattering medium and with the energy window.

A more realistic measurement can be obtained by the use of a 'Phelps phantom' normally consisting of a series of zero activity cylinders placed within a 20 cm diameter uniform flood field (Fig. 3.11). The smallest cylinder visualized can then be used as a guide to the system resolution. The radius of this cylinder is equal to the FWHM which would be obtained by the equivalent system from the measurement of a line source as described above. A

31

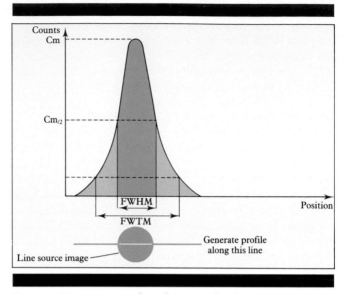

Fig. 3.10 **Measurement of resolution with a line source.**

modification to this phantom is the use of spheres rather than cylinders, in which case the method measures the overall effect of resolution in the reconstructed plane and perpendicular to it (termed slice thickness – see below). However, the results from these measurements are again greatly influenced by the count density in the image; only when clinically realistic values are used will meaningful data be obtained.

The two methods described above are both high contrast evaluations of resolution. The 'Phelps phantom' may be used to obtain low contrast data by placing a different (non-zero) specific activity in the cylinders to that in the flood field and repeating the measurement. Results may be expressed as the minimum contrast at which cylinders of various sizes remain visible in the reconstructed image.

Slice thickness

Slice thickness is the term applied to the system resolution perpendicular to the imaging plane and should not be confused with the linear dimension of the number of pixels

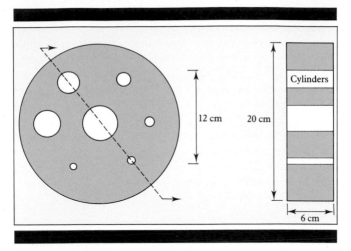

Fig. 3.11 **A 'Phelps phantom'.**

summed together in this direction in a gamma camera system (which is a substantially lower value).

The standard method of measurement is again by the FWHM and FWTM of a line source. However, this time the values for the profile are obtained from consecutive slices of a line source placed parallel to the imaging plane. Different values may again be measured at different points in the field of view and in the presence of scatter.

Another method (which is particularly useful for multi-detector systems) that can produce a different and probably more realistic value is to form the profile from the response to the edge of a flood source (ie as it just moves out of the field of view). The difference is caused first, by the different proportion of scattered radiation present and second, by the different geometry, which is particularly important when focused collimators are used.

Sensitivity

This is usually defined as counts/sec/MBq obtained by the system when imaging a 20 cm long, 20 cm diameter, uniformly filled, perspex cylinder. The result can be affected by the energy resolution of the system and the energy window employed and hence these should be quoted alongside the sensitivity value.

In the case of multi-slice systems it is important to quote the number of slices over which the sensitivity is being summed. Also, misleading results can be obtained for systems which spend some of the scanning time not collecting data (ie step and shoot gamma cameras and the SME). The sensitivity value will probably have been measured using a long acquisition time, and if shorter periods are used clinically then the proportion of the time which is actually used in obtaining data (and hence the effective sensitivity) decreases.

Contrast resolution

If a system is to be used to measure the specific activity at different points in an object then it is necessary not only to visualize the structure but also to reconstruct the correct contrast between different parts of the source. This can be tested using various objects (for example the low contrast 'Phelps phantom' described above) containing a known distribution of specific activity and comparing the true contrast with that obtained in the reconstructed image. It is important to measure contrast recovery throughout the field of view with both small and extended sources of activity. Contrast can be defined in many ways; one suitable measure for an object within a constant background is:

$$\text{Contrast} = \frac{\dfrac{\text{Counts}}{\text{Pixel}} \text{ in object} - \dfrac{\text{Counts}}{\text{Pixel}} \text{ in background}}{\dfrac{\text{Counts}}{\text{Pixel}} \text{ in object} + \dfrac{\text{Counts}}{\text{Pixel}} \text{ in background}}$$

LIMITATIONS OF SPET SYSTEMS

An ideal SPET system would be capable of producing high resolution images in a very short time, allowing high quality dynamic data to be obtained. Unfortunately, due to the relatively low number of gamma photons available for detection, this situation cannot be realized. In choosing a SPET device, careful attention must be paid to the clinical use to which it will be put. In particular the requirement to perform fast dynamic studies may be ruled out either by lack of sensitivity (not allowing sufficient events to be detected in the available time) or by the inability of the detector to complete a data acquisition sequence fast enough (even though it may have sufficient sensitivity). On this subject it is important to distinguish between scanning time (which often refers only to the length of time for which data is collected) and the time it takes to perform the scan (which includes 'redundant' time spent moving the detector while it is not obtaining data). As an example of this, while the SME 810 system is quoted as being able to perform 30-second scans, the actual time with a standard six projection acquisition is in fact approximately 40 seconds. If eighteen projections are required the minimum scanning time is over 2 minutes per slice.

To some extent the sensitivity and resolution of the system can be traded one against another down to a certain minimum resolution. It is, however, important to find how complicated and expensive these changes may be.

Finally, systems are limited to the size of the object which they can scan, but overall count rate (ie count rate response) is seldom, if ever, a problem.

QUALITY CONTROL PROCEDURES

This is a wide field and for detailed descriptions of the methods of performing quality control, the reader should refer to the following references: Jarritt & Cullum 1983, Jarritt & Ell 1984, Keyes 1982, Rogers et al 1981.

Below, the main elements of a quality control program, and why they are necessary, are outlined. In the case of a gamma camera-based system it is also necessary to perform all of the conventional quality control procedures associated with planar scintigraphy (Todd-Pokropek 1980, National Electrical Manufacturers' Association (NEMA) 1980, Hospital Physicists Association (HPA) 1978, Elliot et al 1980, 1982).

Centre of rotation

The data acquired consists of the various projections taken from different angles around the patient. To allow these to be combined to form an image there must be some way of relating a position in one projection with that in another. The way that this is done is from the known angular position of the projection combined with the knowledge of the position at which the image of a point source (or a short line source perpendicular to the imaging plane) appears in each projection. In the case of a non-rotating system (for example the SME 810 using six projections), the position of the source in the field of view is irrelevant, although it is normally placed at, or somewhere near, the centre. However, in a rotating system the source must coincide with the point formed by the intersection of the imaging plane and the line about which the rotation occurs (hence the name 'centre of rotation'). It is important for this point to exist (ie circular motion to occur) and for it to be found accurately (within 1 mm to 2 mm).

Uniformity

Because the final image is formed from a series of projections, it is important that the response, both within, and between, projections is constant. In the ideal system this would be ensured by perfect acquisition hardware; however, in real life this is never the case and corrections have to be made for imperfect responses.

The correction is made using a 'flood source' which presents an identical activity distribution to all of the detectors in a multi-detector system or across the full face of a gamma camera. A correction is calculated for varying sensitivity and this is used to modify the projection data before reconstruction of subsequent images. It is important to realize that the correction factors obtained will be affected by the energy of the isotope, the amount of scatter in the object and the energy window used. Therefore the flood field should contain a realistic amount of scattering material and the isotope and energy window which will be used in subsequent studies should also be used in the calibration.

REFERENCES

Bracewell RN, Riddle AC 1967 Inversion of fan beam scans in radioastronomy. Astrophysics Journal **150**: 429–434
Brooks RA, Di Chiro G 1976 Principles of computer assisted

tomography (CAT) in radiographic and radioisotopic imaging. Physics in Medicine and Biology **21**: 689–732

Budinger TF, Gullberg GT 1974 Three dimensional reconstruction of isotope distributions. Physics in Medicine and Biology **19**: 387–389

Cormack AM 1973 Reconstruction of densities from their projections, with applications in radiological physics. Physics in Medicine and Biology **18**: 195–207

Ell PJ, Deacon JM, Jarritt PH 1980 Atlas of computerized emission tomography. Churchill Livingstone, Edinburgh

Elliot AT, Short MD, Barnes KJ 1980 The performance assessment of gamma cameras. Part 1, Report STB 11/80 DHSS, London

Elliot AT, Short MD, Barnes KJ 1982 The performance assessment of gamma cameras. Part 2. Report STB 13/82, DHSS, London

Gordon R, Bender R, Herman GT 1970 Algebraic reconstruction techniques (ART) for three dimensional electron microscopy and X-ray photography. Journal of Theoretical Biology **29**: 471–481

Herman GT, Rowland S 1971 Resolution in ART; An experimental investigation of the resolving power of an algebraic picture reconstruction technique. Journal of Theoretical Biology **30**: 213–223

Hospital Physicists Association 1978 The theory, specification and testing of Anger type gamma cameras. Task Group Report n.27

Jarritt PH, Cullum ID 1983 Quality control of single photon emission tomographic systems. Quality control of Nuclear Medicine instrumentation. CRS-38: 81–91, HPA, London

Jarritt PH, Ell PJ 1984 Gamma Camera Emission Tomography: Quality Control & Clinical Applications. Current Medical Literature Ltd, London

Kan MK, Hopkins GB 1979 Measurement of liver volume by emission computed tomography. Journal of Nuclear Medicine **20**: 514–520

Kay DB, Keyes JW Jnr., Simon W 1974 Radionuclide tomographic image reconstruction using Fourier transform techniques. Journal of Nuclear Medicine **15**: 981–986

Keyes JW Jnr., Kay DB, Simon W 1973 Digital reconstruction of three dimensional radionuclide images. Journal of

Nuclear Medicine **14:** 628–629

Keyes JW Jnr 1982 Computed Emission Tomography. Oxford University Press

Kemp MC 1980 Maximum entropy reconstructions in emission tomography. International symposium on medical radionuclide imaging. Heidelberg, IAEA SM-247/128

Kuhl DE, Phelps ME, Kowell AP, Metter EJ, Selin C, Winter J 1980 Effects of stroke on local cerebral metabolism and perfusion: Mapping by emission computed tomography of ^{18}FDG and ^{13}NH$_3$. Annals of Neurology **8:** 47–60

Macey DJ, Marshall R 1982 The Lungs. Computed Emission Tomography. Oxford University Press

National Electrical Manufacturers' Association (NEMA) 1980 Standards for performance measurements of scintillation cameras. NEMA, USA

Rogers WL, Clinthorne HH, Harkness BA, Koral KF, Keyes JW Jnr 1981 Flood field requirements for emission computed tomography with an Anger camera. Journal of Nuclear Medicine **23:** 162–168

Shapiro B, Rigby L, Britton KE 1980 The assessment of thyroid volume with single photon emission tomography. Nuclear Medicine Communications **1:** 33–36

Shepp LA, Logan BF 1974 Some insights into the Fourier reconstruction of a head section. IEEE Transactions in Nuclear Science **N21:** 21–43

Todd-Pokropek AE 1980 Specification, acceptance testing and quality control: an outline of some problems in testing gamma camera systems: Nuclear Medicine Communications **1:** 41–48

4 | Data Analysis

In this chapter a brief description of the methods used for analysis of the data available in the CBF-SPET studies, is given.

Analysis of the data is always made in two steps. First, by visual inspection of the data available from the video output of the computer system and second, by quantification of that information. This is based on the regions of interest (ROI) method, applied to the whole-body studies, dynamic gamma camera acquisition and tomographic data, according to protocols that are described in the following sections.

The visual analysis aims to identify patterns of distribution of the radiotracer (^{99m}Tc-HMPAO) in comparison with normal.

QUANTITATIVE ANALYSIS

Whole-body distribution

In whole-body distribution, a regular ROI is drawn around the total body and irregular regions are placed around brain, liver, lungs, heart shadow, bowel loops and urinary bladder. The percentage of uptake (as % of total body) at different time periods is calculated after correction for decay.

Dynamic planar acquisition

In dynamic planar acquisition, regular ROIs are placed on the projection of each common carotid artery and cerebral hemisphere to calculate the variation of radioactivity with time. The time-activity curves are used mainly to study cerebral perfusion of patients with cerebrovascular disease, in particular those with neck vessel disease. The time of peak for the carotid arteries and brain curves may be calculated.

Similar time-activity curve analysis is employed to study the initial (30 minutes) distribution of the tracer throughout the liver, lungs and heart (initially blood-pool, later myocardial uptake).

Single photon emission computerized tomography

The quantitative analysis of SPET data varies according to the particular study undertaken. However, a protocol is applied to the study of patients with dementia of Alzheimer type which may be used for any other study. This is based on the calculation of uptake ratios between the cerebral cortex and the cerebellum. Three methods are used in this book:

1 Method I: general
2 Method II: irregular ROI – % uptake normalized to total slice
3 Method III: regular ROI – ratios of average counts per pixel between cerebrum and cerebellum

Method I: general Three contiguous slices of the cerebellum are summed and the resultant composite image divided into two hemispheres by the midline. Similarly, six to eight slices of the cerebrum are added to form a composite image of the cerebrum, which is divided into two halves by the midline.

A midbrain slice (approximately 25–33 mm above the OM line) containing the basal ganglia is used to draw two horizontal lines perpendicular to the midline, one above the most anterior part of the heads of the caudate nuclei, the other below the most posterior part of the thalami (Fig. 4.1).

Two ROI for the cerebellum (right and left) and six ROI for the cerebrum (anterior, middle and posterior for each hemisphere) are then created following the contours of the composite images and the lines. These ROI correspond respectively to the frontal lobe (anterior), the parieto-temporal lobes (middle) and parieto-occipital lobes (posterior). They permit the calculation of total activity,

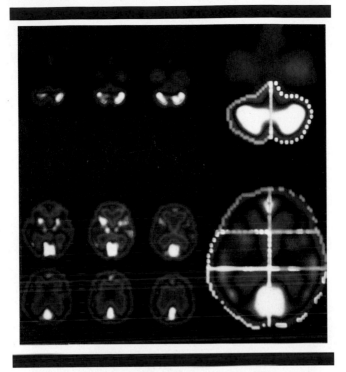

Fig. 4.1 **ROIs used in Method I for quantitative analysis of SPET data.**

average counts per pixel and percentage of tracer uptake on those different areas of the brain.

This method reveals only gross abnormalities. It cannot separate grey from white matter perfusion deficits. In addition it is impossible to discriminate small structural changes due to the dilution in a large sampling area of the brain.

This general quantitative approach has been used to study changes in tracer uptake/retention in the brain induced by CO_2 (Choksey et al 1989).

Method II: irregular ROI – % uptake normalized to total slice This method is designed to study changes of tracer uptake in the basal ganglia of patients with Parkinson's disease. These patients have movement disorders that make

their positioning very difficult and they require relatively
fast data acquisition protocols. Some do not tolerate an
acquisition period as long as the 35 minutes taken with the
conventional rotating gamma camera. The single slice
tomographic brain scanner can then be of paramount
importance. However, it is not always possible to obtain a
total set of slices of the entire brain. In some cases only two
contiguous slices are acquired.

To maintain the analysis protocol constant for these
particular patients, irregular ROI are drawn around the
basal ganglia (head of the caudate nucleus, putamen/globus
palidus and thalamus) and the contour of the total slice, as
seen in Figure 4.2.

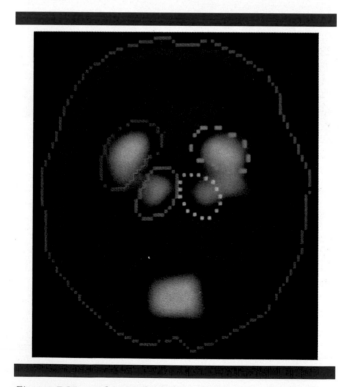

Fig. 4.2 **ROIs used in Method II for quantitative analysis of
SPET data.**

The % uptake in each structure (ROI) is then calculated as follows:

(total counts in ROI/total counts in slice) × 100

This final result is afterwards averaged for the two contiguous slices, containing the basal ganglia.

Method III: regular ROI – average counts per pixel This is a more discriminative method. Regular ROI of 4 × 4 pixels (128 × 128 matrix resolution) are used on slices of two pixel width. The majority of the clinical work presented in this book was performed with the IGE 400AC/STARCAM. In this system each pixel (128 × 128 matrix resolution) is 3.3 mm × 3.3 mm. Therefore, one voxel (4 × 4 × 2 pixels) corresponds to brain tissue samples of approximately 1.15 cm^3. This value is within the resolution capability of the instrument (FWHM = 10 mm) as tested with the 'Phelps phantom'.

Samples of different cerebral cortex areas and cerebellum are obtained from at least three contiguous slices (Costa et al 1986). On each slice two, three or more samples for each area on each side are collected (Fig. 4.3). The samples from the cerebellum on each side are averaged and the process is repeated for the different cerebral cortex areas.

The activity ratio between each cortical area (average counts per voxel) and the cerebellar hemisphere with higher average counts per voxel is calculated. Although defined for cerebral cortex areas, this method may be used for any brain structure.

The cerebellum is often used in these studies as a reference structure. This is because the cerebellum is often relatively uninvolved, when compared with all the other grey and white matter structures in the brain. However it is of course possible to use other areas of the brain for reference, such as the occipital visual cortex or even the basal ganglia. Protocols can then be optimized, if one considers specific pathologic conditions (cross cerebellar diaschisis, alcoholic dementia, movement disorders, etc.).

DISTRIBUTION OF ^{99M}Tc-HMPAO IN NORMAL MAN

Immediately after the intravenous injection, ^{99m}Tc-HMPAO

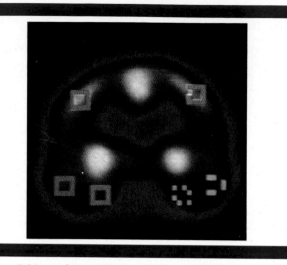

Fig. 4.3 **ROIs used in Method III for quantitative analysis of SPET data.**

is distributed throughout the whole body according to the distribution of the cardiac output and regional blood flow. However, the amount of tracer available for extraction by the different organs is reduced due to its binding to blood cells (Costa et al 1986, Ell et al 1986, Sharp et al 1986) and to proteins in the plasma (Costa et al 1986).

The final regional distribution of this tracer depends on the uptake and retention mechanism in different organs. The total body retention of ^{99m}Tc-HMPAO at 24 hours post-injection is 68% (measured with a whole-body counter) and its total urinary excretion at the same time is 38% (measured in urine samples, Costa et al 1986).

Whole-body distribution
The extraction of ^{99m}Tc-HMPAO (3 hours post-injection) by different organs of a normal individual is shown in Figure 4.4.

Head and neck The brain is well differentiated from the surrounding background activity of facial and extracranial blood-pool. There is a faint demonstration of the salivary

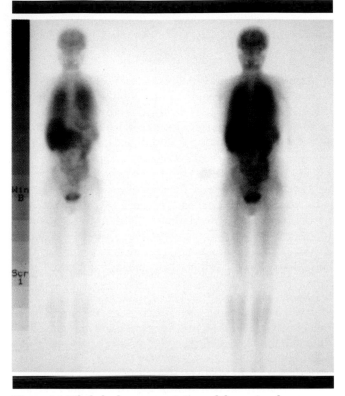

Figure 4.4 **Whole-body representation of the regional distribution of 99mTc-HMPAO. The image on the right-hand side is a darker display to facilitate the visualization of the 99mTc-HMPAO uptake in the soft tissue, particularly the skeletal muscles of the calves and thighs.**

glands and secretory mucosa of the mouth and nose. Skeletal muscle is well visualized (tongue and masseter).

In the rest of the body there is a generalized small background activity due to tracer present in the blood-pool of the soft tissues (mainly subcutaneous adipose tissue).

Thorax Both lungs are well seen, as is the myocardium. In females the breasts are faintly shown with an activity slightly higher than the background. In the thorax this background activity is increased in people with large amounts of adipose tissue and much more in those subjects with large skeletal muscle masses.

Abdomen ^{99m}Tc-HMPAO is excreted in significant amounts by the liver and the hepatobiliary system which carries the tracer into the bowel loops (always seen as early as 20 minutes post-injection). The spleen is well demonstrated, probably due to its high blood-pool. The urinary bladder is always clearly visualized, demonstrating the urinary excretion of the compound. The kidneys are not well seen unless there is a degree of renal obstruction.

In females, the uterus can be sometimes demonstrated, unless obscured by the bladder.

Limbs The vein proximal to the site of injection is invariably observed with different degrees of tracer retention even if the injection technique is followed by a careful wash through with saline. The skeletal muscles are unusually well demonstrated and with intensity of tracer deposition clearly higher than in adipose tissue. This enables the differentiation between skeletal muscle and fat, especially in the buttocks where some authors had misinterpreted the distribution of the ^{99m}Tc-HMPAO (Sharp et al 1986). (The intense activity shown in the area of the buttocks and inner thighs by these authors is not fat but skeletal muscle.) In fact, an important characteristic of the *d,l* isomer of ^{99m}Tc-HMPAO is that its uptake/retention in skeletal muscles is well differentiated from the background blood-pool activity in adipose tissue.

Distribution changes with time

Whole-body images obtained at 20, 45 and 60 minutes and at 2.5 hours post-injection of the tracer reveal that there is good brain retention with no significant change in the brain uptake during the first hour (Table 4.1).

Excretion of ^{99m}Tc-HMPAO in man is seen to be via the hepatobiliary (into the bowel) and urinary systems. The lung extraction of ^{99m}Tc-HMPAO is relatively high and appears to vary according to lung pathology (El-Gazzar

Table 4.1 **Regional body distribution of ^{99m}Tc-HMPAO in man. Results are expressed as % of total dose administered.**

Organ	Time post-injection			
	20 min	45 min	60 min	2.5 hrs
Brain	6.1	6.2	6.1	5.5
Lungs	14.5	13.8	13.3	11.2
Liver	23.7	22.4	21.3	17.5
Gut	22.4	23.2	24.1	26.3
Urinary bladder	6.7	8.9	10.4	19.4

et al 1987). Initial observations show that there is a slightly higher lung extraction by smokers.

Blood clearance and distribution

The blood clearance of ^{99m}Tc-HMPAO (3.7 MBq) in a normal subject determined from 10 ml blood samples collected at 3, 7, 14, 30 minutes, and at 1, 2 and 5 hours post injection is shown in Figure 4.5. The majority of the tracer is extracted from the circulation during the first 20–30 minutes post-injection, most rapidly between the first two data points (3 and 7 minutes). This is also seen with time-activity curve analysis obtained from a ROI over the heart following dynamic planar acquisition with a gamma camera. There is an initial, very rapid, transit with a $t_{\frac{1}{2}}$ of 3 seconds, from the peak (9–11 seconds), followed by a second component ($t_{\frac{1}{2}} = 36$ seconds) and a slower component with a $t_{\frac{1}{2}}$ of approximately 8 minutes, between 5 and 30 minutes post-injection (Costa et al 1986).

The distribution of ^{99m}Tc-HMPAO between blood cells and plasma shows a higher partition to the plasma fraction during the first 60 minutes post-injection (approximately 55%). At 5 hours, and particularly at 24 hours, this predominance is reversed, with more tracer bound to blood cells (53 and 67% respectively). This is clearly demonstrated in Figure 4.6.

It is apparent that after 5 hours post-injection the rate of excretion of the radiotracer from the plasma is increased, while that from the blood cells is reduced. It is unlikely that red cells, white cells and platelets accumulate tracer between 5 and 24 hours since by this time the tracer is

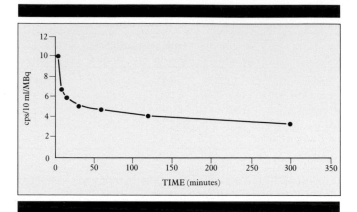

Fig. 4.5 **⁹⁹ᵐTc-HMPAO clearance from total blood.**

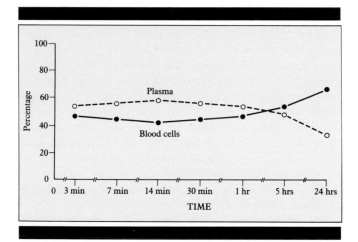

Fig. 4.6 **Distribution of ⁹⁹ᵐTc-HMPAO between plasma and blood cells.**

bound to plasma proteins and no longer available in its lipophilic form. Figure 4.7 illustrates the more rapid clearance from the plasma after 5 hours. The fall between 2 and 5 hours probably indicates either excretion of the protein-bound fraction or its breakdown into more hydrophilic molecules which are removed from the circulation.

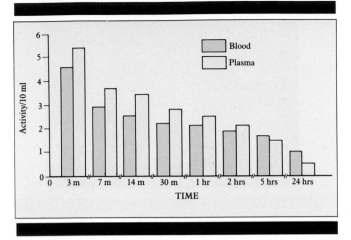

Fig. 4.7 ^{99m}Tc-HMPAO clearance from plasma and blood cells.

Regional brain distribution

Immediately after intravenous injection and circulation through the pulmonary vascular bed the tracer is deposited in the brain during the first passage through the cerebral circulation (Costa et al 1986). In normal circumstances, uptake/retention of ^{99m}Tc-HMPAO follows the distribution of the rCBF and permits the differentiation between grey matter and white matter.

Areas of expected higher flow rates are shown (Fig. 4.8) with more intense deposition of ^{99m}Tc-HMPAO (eg visual cortex, basal ganglia, thalamus, apart from cerebellum) than the rest of the brain cortex.

The cortex of frontal, parietal, temporal and occipital lobes shows areas of variable intensity of tracer uptake reflecting local anatomy and functional differentiation. In normals, rCBF and metabolism follow a parallel (coupled) course. The lateral ventricles are seldom seen well differentiated from the surrounding peri-ventricular white matter. This reflects the limitation of the method in the resolution of the smaller structures of the brain. However, it is possible to identify enlargement of the lateral ventricles (Fig. 4.9) whenever the space between the head of the caudate nuclei is greater than normal.

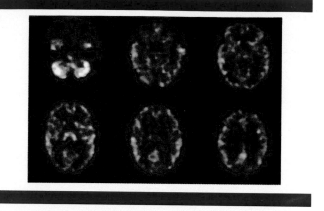

Fig. 4.8 **Normal perfusion pattern. Six transverse slices (parallel to the OM line) obtained with the SME 810 brain scanner from an individual with no intracranial pathology. The cerebellum (top left), temporal lobes (top middle), frontal and temporal cortex (top right), subcortical structures – head of caudate nucleus, putamen/globus pallidus, thalamus – and visual cortex (bottom left), and frontal and parietal cortex (bottom middle and right) are clearly identified.**

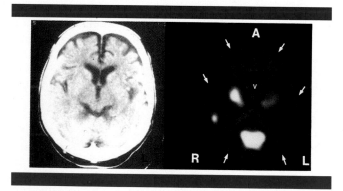

Fig. 4.9 **Enlargement of lateral ventricles in a patient with Alzheimer's disease. The small arrows point to cortical areas with severely impaired perfusion, more severe than the cortical atrophy seen with X-ray CT scanning. V-enlarged lateral ventricles; A-anterior; R-right; L-left.**

REFERENCES

Choksey MS, Costa DC, Iannotti I, Ell PJ, Crockard HA 1989 ^{99m}Tc-HMPAO SPET and cerebral blood flow: a study of CO_2 reactivity. Nuclear Medicine Communications 10: 609–618

Costa DC, Ell PJ, Cullum ID, Jarritt PH 1986 The *in vivo* distribution of ^{99m}Tc-HMPAO in normal man. Nuclear Medicine Communications 7: 647–658

El-Gazzar AH, Sadek S, Bahar R, Rageb A, Omar YT, Abdel-Dayem HM 1987 Uptake of ^{99m}Tc-Hexamethylpropylene-amineoxime (^{99m}Tc-HMPAO) by healthy and diseased lungs. Nuclear Medicine 26: 149–190

Ell PJ, Hocknell JML, Costa DC, et al 1986 ^{99m}Tc-Hexamethyl-propyleneamineoxime (^{99m}Tc-HMPAO): a breakthrough in radionuclide CBF tomography. Nuklearmedizin, Suppl. 22: S179–S181

Sharp PF, Smith FW, Gemmell HG, et al 1986 Technetium-99m-HMPAO stereoisomers as potential agents for imaging regional cerebral blood flow: human volunteer studies. Journal of Nuclear Medicine 27: 171–177

TRANSVERSE SECTIONS

Transverse slices of a normal rCBF SPET with HMPAO are compared side by side with post-mortem transverse sections (2.5 cm thick) from the brain of a 75-year-old male who died (suddenly) of a ruptured dissecting aneurysm of the aorta. There was no gross structural abnormality. A small degree of cortical atrophy (age-related) was observed. Figure 5.1 A–D illustrates comparative anatomy of the brain and perfusion maps in transverse sections.

CORONAL SECTIONS

Coronal slices obtained with the rotating gamma camera (IGE 400AC/STARCAM) are compared with coronal sections (2.5 cm thick) of another post-mortem human

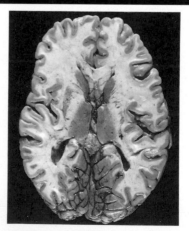

(A)

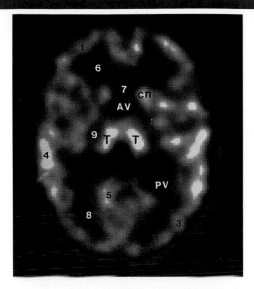

(B)

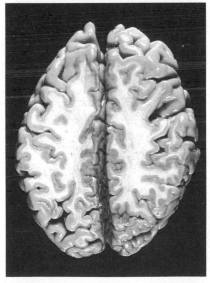

(C)

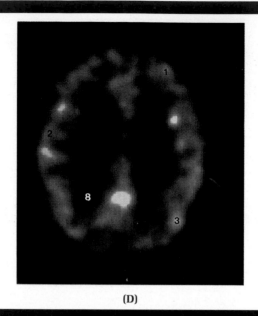

(D)

Fig. 5.1 **A–D Comparison between anatomy (from post-mortem specimen) and perfusion maps in transverse sections. Key: 1–frontal cortex; 2–parietal cortex; 3–posterior parietal cortex; 4–temporal cortex (m–mesial; l–lateral); 5–visual cortex; 6–frontal lobe white matter; 7–corpus callosum; 8–white matter of the parietal and occipital lobes; 9–internal capsule; AV–anterior horns of the lateral ventricles; PV–posterior horns of the lateral ventricles; cn–head of the caudate nucleus; T–thalamus.**

brain, a 58-year-old female with ischaemic heart disease who died from an acute myocardial infarction. The brain showed no structural abnormality in either the grey matter or white matter. Figure 5.2 A–D illustrates comparative anatomy and perfusion maps.

VISUAL INTERPRETATION OF SPET IMAGES

Important features

The interpretation of rCBF SPET maps is helped by a

detailed knowledge of anatomy of the brain and its cortical and subcortical structures known to have distinct perfusion patterns. These maps should be studied in different planes of orientation, which enable a better identification of lesions and individualization of the different areas of the brain. Whenever possible, transverse (parallel to the OM line), reorientated coronal (perpendicular to transverse) and of less importance, sagittal sections should be analysed.

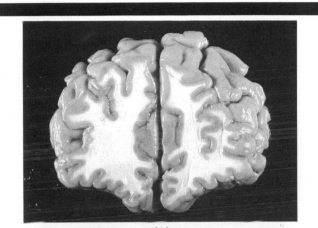

(A)

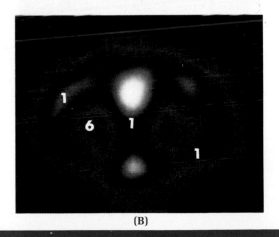

(B)

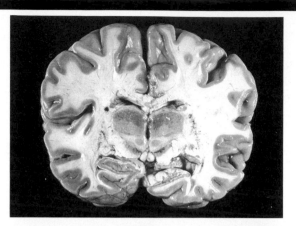

(C)

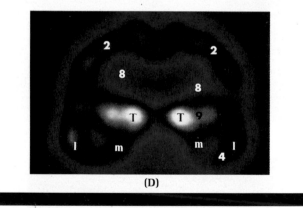

(D)

Fig. 5.2 **A–D Comparison between anatomy (from post-mortem specimen) and perfusion maps in coronal slices obtained with gamma camera. For key, refer to Fig. 5.1.**

A colour display needs to be chosen according to the preference of the observer and maintained unaltered. This permits a more reliable representation of the tomographic maps. Several important points need to be carefully considered for the visual interpretation of rCBF SPET maps:

1   The shape of the brain image and contours for each slice

2   The homogeneity of ^{99m}Tc-HMPAO distribution, paying attention to the filter characteristics used during reconstruction (small vessel disease produces usually a very heterogenous perfusion pattern due to the irregularity of distribution of the tracer throughout the brain structures)

3   The identification of the different cortical areas (frontal, superior parietal, posterior parietal, mesial temporal, lateral temporal, occipital), subcortical structures (head of the caudate nucleus, putamen/globus pallidus, thalamus), brain stem and cerebellum for both hemispheres

4   White matter structures are usually identified as areas of low tracer concentration lying between the head of the caudate nucleus, putamen/globus pallidus and thalamus (internal and external capsula)

5   The peri-ventricular white matter is usually difficult to separate from the lateral ventricles

6   The ventricular space lies between the heads of the caudate nuclei and the outer areas of low tracer concentration correspond to the peri-ventricular white matter, so that dilated ventricles give an appearance of widening of the space between the heads of the caudate nuclei

7   Coronal sections help to differentiate between the mesial and the lateral cortex of the temporal lobes and help to visualize better the superior frontal and the superior parietal cortex, particularly the areas close to the midline, around the inter-hemispheric groove

8   Sagittal slices allow for a single comparison to be made in the same section, between frontal, parietal, occipital lobes and cerebellum

9   Identification of asymmetries between hemispheres is a relatively easy task which should always be confirmed by quantitative analysis. A difference of more than 5% is abnormal

10 Relative quantification of areas of relative decrease or increase of tracer concentration is helpful

MIGRAINE

Headache is a common symptom, frequently taken as a trivial disorder, but it may sometimes be a sign of severe disease. The pathology behind each type of headache varies from scalp lesions due to trauma or stress (tension headache produced by hypertonic muscles of neck and scalp) to intracranial space-occupying lesions (tumours).

Changes in the calibre and permeability of cranial arteries and veins may produce headache. This has been thought of as one of the mechanisms responsible for the development of migraine attacks. According to this vascular theory (Wolff 1963), vasoconstriction of cerebral arteries leads to neurological symptoms (aura, paraesthesiae), while rebound vasodilatation of either extra-or intracranial vessels causes the headache.

Aetiology

The aetiology of migraine is complex and because it is not a fatal disease, pathologic observations are rare. Therefore there is a need to better understand the neuropathologic mechanisms involved in migraine. Differential diagnosis of migraine is based upon criteria defined by Vahlquist (1955). Two main types of migraine can be easily distinguished, *classical migraine* (focal neurological symptoms always present, preceded by an aura), and *common migraine* (headache without focal neurological symptoms). The difference between the two suggests that causative events during an acute attack of classical migraine are distinct from common migraine. In fact, the majority of reports on common migraine failed to demonstrate any significant change in rCBF as Lauritzen & Olesen (1984) have shown with the ^{133}Xe inhalation technique and SPET. On the other hand, they reported that 8 of their 11 patients with classical migraine exhibited areas of cortical hypoperfusion concordant with the clinical presentation (focal neurological symptoms) during the attack. Those patients studied during an asymptomatic period after treatment showed variable patterns of perfusion in the tomographic ^{133}Xe-rCBF maps. Some revealed no interhemispheric asymmetry, while others showed persistent hypoperfusion, either similar or less marked than in the first study. These findings are in agreement with previous work by Olesen and co-workers (1981a) who never found any area of hyperperfusion during the headache phase of induced acute attacks of classical migraine.

With ^{133}Xe-rCBF tomography the average reduction of cortical rCBF (17%) was less marked than that determined with the two-dimensional multi-probe method (24%). Lauritzen & Olesen (1984) attributed this discrepancy to technical limitations due to the super-imposition of brain structures in the two-dimensional method and increased Compton-scatter from the surrounding brain tissue with SPET. However, there was a consistent finding of hypoperfused areas (unilateral or bilateral), mainly in the posterior part of the brain (posterior parietal, temporal and occipital cortex). Only one patient showed hypoperfusion confined to the frontal cortex. Three patients showed no significant change in rCBF during the induction of the attack of classical migraine. The authors stated that this might be due to a reversal of rCBF changes by the time of ^{133}Xe-SPET study. Two of their patients restudied after recovery (one spontaneous remission and the other after treatment) showed hyperperfusion of the previously hypoperfused cortical areas.

That hypoperfusion may represent a dynamic process, is reinforced by the events described during the 'Leão's spreading depression' (Leão 1944). A moderate cortical hypoperfusion persists for hours, spreading slowly through the cerebral cortex and is probably caused by a local disturbance of the vasomotor regulation. This might reflect an initial disturbance in the brain metabolism which causes the symptoms and evokes secondary vasomotor changes. It was hoped that ^{99m}Tc-HMPAO and high resolution SPET might demonstrate similar changes. In addition, SPET might help to identify subcortical abnormalities never found by previous workers. Only Lauritzen & Olesen (1984) briefly refer to small asymmetries of ^{133}Xe-rCBF-SPET in these brain structures. However, their technique lacks enough spatial and contrast resolution, and partial volume effect is severely augmented by the low photon energy of ^{133}Xe.

SPET investigations

In collaboration with the Academic Unit of Neurosciences, Charing Cross and Westminster Medical School, and the Department of Nuclear Medicine, Charing Cross Hospital, a series of 38 patients with different types of headache were studied, using ^{99m}Tc-HMPAO and SPET (Costa et al 1988a).

Patients   14 males and 24 females with an age range from 23 to 69 years were investigated. Vahlquist's criteria were used to distinguish between classical and common migraine. In addition, patients with tension headache and cluster headache were studied for comparison. The following list shows the distribution of patients according to their type of headache:

Type of headache	No. of patients
Classical migraine	14
Common migraine	9
Tension headache	12
Cluster headache	3

All the patients with migraine were investigated during a spontaneous acute attack (aura or headache phase) at different times after the onset; 3 of the 13 classical migraine and 3 of the 9 common migraine patients had repeat studies when asymptomatic.

Regional brain distribution of ^{99m}Tc-HMPAO   The high resolution of the investigations performed with the SME 810 tomographic scanner permits the identification of deep subcortical structures, as well as the distinction between grey matter and white matter from the cerebrum. In addition, it enables the identification of extra-cranial perfusion (mainly temporal muscles) well separated from the brain.

The majority of studies showed no major perfusion abnormality within the regional distribution of ^{99m}Tc-HMPAO in the cortex and subcortical areas of the brain. No consistent pattern emerged for the identification of any of the categories of patients. Nevertheless, changes in the perfusion patterns were found in several patients.

A. *Classical migraine* Four of the 13 classical migraineurs had decreased perfusion in the posterior parieto-temporal areas, always unilateral and corresponding to the focal neurological symptoms. These seem to agree with previous work with ^{133}Xe-rCBF-SPET (Lauritzen & Olesen 1984). X-ray CT scan, performed whenever patient consent could be obtained, showed no structural abnormality corresponding to the area of decreased perfusion.

The three individuals studied when asymptomatic showed only a slight change in the cortical perfusion compared to the first study. One of them investigated during the aura phase (left visual aura) of the spontaneous acute attack of classical migraine had a small area compatible with deficient perfusion in the right mesial occipital cortex, corresponding to the visual cortical representation. Two weeks later a repeat investigation demonstrated the same area of underperfusion in the right visual cortex, less marked than in the first study during the aura phase (shown by the small arrows in Fig. 6.1).

Small asymmetry of the tracer uptake in the heads of the caudate nucleus (right lower than left) was observed in 5 of 9 patients with unilateral headache during the acute attack. This asymmetry was always greater than 5%, and with lower perfusion ipsilateral to the side of pain. Occasionally, underperfusion of the mesial cortex of the temporal lobes can also be seen.

One classical migraine patient was studied for more than 5 hours into the headache phase of a spontaneous acute attack. The ^{99m}Tc-HMPAO-SPET study showed hyperperfusion in the right frontal cortex with no other significant abnormality. Although isolated in this series,

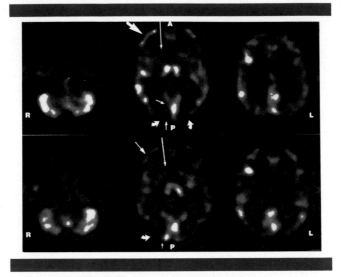

Fig. 6.1 ⁹⁹ᵐTc-HMPAO-SPET maps of a patient with classical migraine during the aura phase (top row) of a spontaneous attack and (two weeks later) when he was asymptomatic (bottom row). The thin long arrow points to the lower perfusion in the right head of the caudate nucleus which improved in the asymptomatic study.

this finding has been observed by Andersen et al (1988) using the inhalation ¹³³Xe-rCBF-SPET method. This author reported that in seven patients with classical migraine, hyperaemia, lasting for 1 to 24 hours, was found a long time after the resolution of the aura phase.

B. *Common migraine* Two of the nine common migraine patients showed decreased perfusion in the posterior parieto-occipital cortex, bilateral and symmetrical (shown by the arrows in Fig. 6.2). The main visual cortex appeared always with preserved perfusion. These findings showed no change when repeat studies were carried out more than three weeks later. Those bilateral and symmetrical parieto-occipital perfusion deficits may be normal variants, which would be in keeping with the normal rCBF values encountered by Olesen et al (1981b) and by Lauritzen &

Olesen (1984) with ^{133}Xe-rCBF-SPET studies of patients during respectively induced and spontaneous attacks of common migraine. However, asymmetries of the rCBF were observed by Levine et al (1987) with ^{133}Xe planar studies using an eight probe pairs home-built instrument.

In 5 of 7 common migraineurs with unilateral headache there was asymmetry of the tracer uptake in the head of the caudate nucleus (4 right lower than left; 1 left lower than right). The hypoperfused nucleus was ipsilateral to the side of headache as seen with studies of patients with classical migraine.

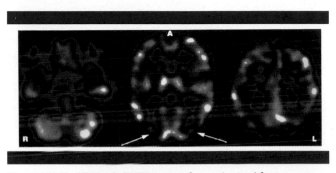

Fig. 6.2 ^{99m}Tc-HMPAO-SPET maps of a patient with common migraine during the headache phase of a spontaneous acute attack.

C. *Tension headache* All studies of patients with tension headache showed uptake in the temporal muscles well separated from the intracranial structures. In 2 of the 12 tension headache sufferers this was abnormally high (Fig. 6.3).

However, this was, by no means, characteristic of this group of patients. Although less intense, similar changes were found in the other categories of patients, either during the headache period study (4 classical, 7 common migraineurs) or in the asymptomatic study (2 classical and 1 common migraine patients). The three patients with cluster headache showed a minor degree of temporal muscle uptake, similar to that seen in normal individuals.

D. *Cluster headache* The three patients investigated showed

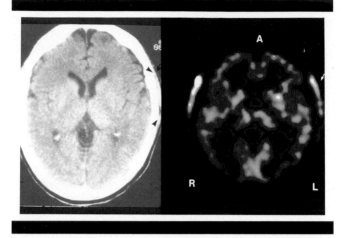

Fig. 6.3 ⁹⁹ᵐTc-HMPAO-SPET maps of a patient with tension headache. Intense tracer concentration is seen in the temporal muscles, bilaterally. X-ray CT scanning is shown on the left for comparison.

a normal pattern of regional distribution of ⁹⁹ᵐTc-HMPAO in the cortical and subcortical structures.

Conclusion

⁹⁹ᵐTc-HMPAO and SPET can demonstrate changes in the perfusion of the cortex and subcortical structures in the brain of some patients with different headache syndromes. These are, however, not consistent.

Cortical hypoperfusion seems more frequent in classical migraine subjects, and some individuals with tension headache show more marked extracranial temporal muscle uptake. The variability of findings in classical migraine may be explained by the wide range of time scale of studies. Because all individuals were investigated during spontaneous acute attacks, ⁹⁹ᵐTc-HMPAO-SPET studies were carried out at different times post onset of symptoms.

PARKINSON'S DISEASE

Parkinson's disease or Paralysis agitans, named after James Parkinson, who first described this clinical condition in

1817, is the most common form of Parkinsonian syndrome. This syndrome is defined as a disturbance of motor function characterized by slowing of emotions and voluntary movements, akinesia, muscular rigidity and tremor.

Aetiology

Parkinsonism, as it is frequently called, is caused by lesions in the substantia nigra and its efferent pathways (Walton 1985). However, it may be produced by several different pathologic processes. The most frequent change is degeneration of the pigmented, dopaminergic neurons of the substantia nigra and adjacent midbrain (Hornykiewicz 1972). In addition, loss of dopaminergic (non-nigral pigmented) neurons in the ventral tegmental area, the source of the mesolimbic-mesocortical dopaminergic system, was described by Uhl et al (1985). These lesions lead to a severe loss of dopamine concentration, mainly in the caudate nucleus and putamen, which presumably initiates the motor disorders of Parkinson's disease.

L-dopa (levodopa) has been used for the treatment (Muenter & Tyce 1971), in an attempt to re-establish dopamine levels and improve motor performance of patients with Parkinson's disease. After 10 years of experience with levodopa therapy, over 50% of patients develop random fluctuations of their motor performance (Marsden & Parkes 1976). Some fluctuations are related to the time of drug administration. Dyskinetic disorders occur when plasma levels of levodopa are rising or falling, with satisfactory motor performance during peak plasma levels. However, there are patients who experience rapid changes between mobility and complete immobility with no relation to the drug administration (the 'ON-OFF syndrome'). These patients with 'ON-OFF' fluctuations are rather therapy-dependent (Nutt et al 1984).

Although the relationships between levodopa administration, plasma concentration, brain levels of the drug and clinical response are not clear, changes in rCBF and oxygen metabolism, studied with PET, have been reported in the basal ganglia and frontal cortex of patients with Parkinson's disease (Wolfson et al 1985). Leenders et al (1985) demonstrated that in clinically effective doses, acute oral administration of L-dopa increases the mean rCBF by 13% in the cerebral cortex and by 20% in the basal ganglia.

SPET investigations

^{99m}Tc-HMPAO-SPET changes in patients with the 'ON-OFF' syndrome of Parkinson's disease, and their relationship with levodopa treatment withdrawal are now described. There is a focus on changes in the basal ganglia, particularly in the head of the caudate nucleus and thalamus, since these seem to be the structures most frequently involved. Cortical changes appear to be secondary.

Patients Ten Parkinson's disease patients (8 male, 2 female) with an age range from 48 to 72 years old and oscillating clinical response to levodopa therapy ('ON-OFF' syndrome) were investigated twice:

1 During an 'ON' phase (on treatment with levodopa)
2 A repeat ^{99m}Tc-HMPAO-SPET investigation after levodopa withdrawal to evoke an 'OFF' phase

The Hoehn and Yarh scale was used to grade the patients' clinical situation. This considers five different grades according to the motor performance at each stage:

I.   Unilateral involvement only, minimal or no functional impairment.
II.   Bilateral or midline involvement, without impairment of balance.
III. First sign of impaired reflexes. Unsteadiness as patient turns or when pushed from standing equilibrium. Functionally restricted, but may have some work potential. Physically capable of leading independent life; disability mild to moderate.
IV.   Fully developed, severely disabling disease; still able to walk and stand unassisted, but markedly incapacitated.
V.   Confined to bed or wheelchair unless aided.

None of the patients presented with stage I. All patients suffered a significant aggravation of their stage when levodopa was withdrawn. The maintenance dose of levodopa ranged from 500 to 1100 mg per day. The repeat study was always carried out as soon as patients showed their characteristic signs of 'OFF' phase after avoiding the first dose fraction of the day. Three patients were studied with the SME 810 dedicated tomographic brain scanner and the other seven with the IGE 400AC/STARCAM system. Data analysis was performed using methods I and II described previously (see pp. 40–41)

^{99m}Tc-HMPAO distribution in cerebral cortex

A. *Visual analysis* The distribution of the tracer is irregular with a variety of non-specific perfusion patterns. Areas of more severe perfusion deficits are usually observed in the frontal, parietal and posterior parietal cortex. These are more marked 'OFF' levodopa than when patients are in

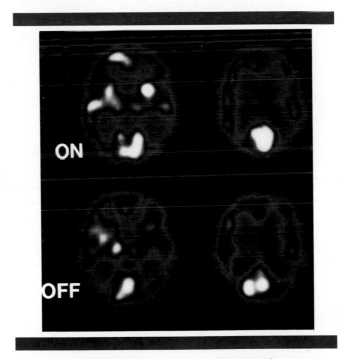

Fig. 6.4 ^{99m}Tc-HMPAO-SPET maps of a patient with Parkinson's disease 'ON' and 'OFF' levodopa obtained with a rotating gamma camera.

control of their voluntary movements ('ON' phase). Figure 6.4 demonstrates that during the 'OFF' levodopa phase there is further impairment of the deficit in perfusion seen in the frontal, high parietal and posterior parietal cortex. In addition there are also significant changes of perfusion seen in the basal ganglia (caudate nucleus and putamen/ globus pallidus) as well as in the thalamus. These abnormalities are better displayed in Fig. 6.5, taken from a study undertaken with the SME 810 tomographic brain scanner. This clearly shows that from 'ON' to 'OFF' there is a decrease in the ^{99m}Tc-HMPAO concentration in the basal ganglia, both the caudate nucleus and the complex putamen/globus pallidus, while there is an increase in the thalamus.

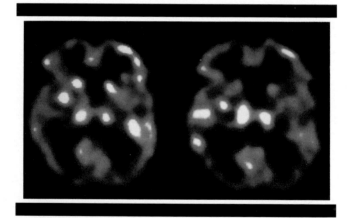

Fig. 6.5 **SME 810 ^{99m}Tc-HMPAO-SPET maps of a patient with Parkinson's disease 'ON' and 'OFF' levodopa. Tracer concentration in the heads of the caudate nuclei drops when patient is 'OFF' levodopa. The opposite is seen in the thalami.**

B. *Quantitative analysis* Quantitative data analysis confirmed the visual findings. There was no significant difference in the lateralisation (L/R) and grey matter over white matter (G/W) ratios between 'ON' and 'OFF' levodopa phases. Individual ratios are shown in Table 6.1; comparison between 'ON' and 'OFF' phases was carried out using the students' t test for paired samples.

Table 6.1 **Left (L) over right (R) and grey (G) over white (W) matter ratios in patients with the 'ON-OFF' syndrome of Parkinson's' disease**

| | L/R | | G/W | |
	'ON'	'OFF'	'ON'	'OFF'
Patient 1	0.99	0.99	1.50	1.97
Patient 2	0.97	0.97	1.87	1.76
Patient 3	1.06	1.07	1.76	1.84
Patient 4	0.99	1.01	2.03	2.06
Patient 5	0.98	0.94	1.64	1.93
Patient 6	0.98	1.01	1.65	1.76
Patient 7	0.99	1.03	1.59	1.61
Patient 8	1.08	1.09	1.48	1.56
Patient 9	1.08	1.04	1.45	1.55
Patient 10	1.02	0.99	1.62	1.61
Mean	1.01	1.01	1.66	1.77
1SD	0.04	0.04	0.17	0.17
Student's t test (paired samples)	$p = 1.000$		$p = 0.069$	

Figure 6.6 shows the changes in the concentration of ^{99m}Tc-HMPAO in the caudate nucleus (as a representative structure of the basal ganglia) and thalamus. The percentage of change is calculated as follows:

$$\Delta\% = [(OFF - ON)/(OFF + ON)/2] \times 100$$

The average decrease in the caudate nucleus uptake is −23.13% and −32.50%, respectively, for the right and left hemispheres. On the other hand, the uptake in the thalamus increases +14.38% (right) and +14.27% (left). The changes in the caudate nucleus are consistent with previous PET studies by Leenders et al (1985) who found an increase in the rCBF of basal ganglia after the administration of L-dopa. The same group (Wolfson et al 1985) found a significant increase in the rCBF of basal ganglia of patients with bilateral Parkinson's disease after the administration of a mixture of L-dopa and carbidopa (Sinemet®). This was not accompanied by any significant change in the regional cerebral metabolic rate of oxygen (rCMRO$_2$). However, Leenders et al (1985) reported a small decrease of the

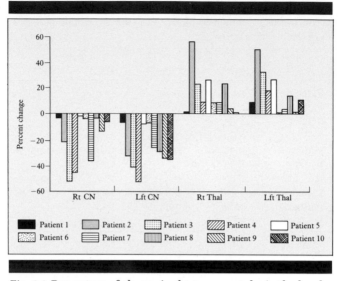

Fig. 6.6 **Percentage of change in the tracer uptake in the head of the caudate nucleus and thalamus.**

rCMRO$_2$ (2.0 – 4.6%), respectively in the cortex and basal ganglia) after acute administration of L-dopa. These authors consider this evidence of the direct vasodilator effects of L-dopa and not a response to regional metabolic demands. Nevertheless, animal studies have shown that levodopa produces a regional increase of the glucose utilization in the motor nuclei and hypothalamus of rats (Warner et al 1982). There may therefore be regional differences that may be observed only if high resolution imaging techniques are used.

In the present studies, either with a gamma camera or dedicated tomographic brain scanner, the spatial resolution (around 9 to 10 mm FWHM) allows for the separation of the head of the caudate nucleus from the complex putamen/globus pallidus and the clear individualization of the thalamus. Whether the changes encountered in the caudate nucleus (decreased perfusion after levodopa withdrawal) are purely rCBF-dependent or due to other causes remains unexplained. The same applies to the changes seen in cortical perfusion. Even more difficult to explain are the changes in the opposite direction observed in the thalamus. If ^{99m}Tc-HMPAO reflects only the distribution of rCBF, then the changes encountered should be always in the same direction for the different structures studied, with single values dependent on the regional differences in levodopa concentration and amplitude of vasodilator response.

Three possible explanations for the reduction in the relative perfusion of the head of caudate nucleus and increase in the perfusion of the thalamus may be proposed. First, the total amount of ^{99m}Tc-HMPAO in the brain section studied and in the caudate nucleus after levodopa withdrawal may have decreased much more than the tracer in the thalamus. This would give higher thalamic concentrations (relative to total slice), particularly if the decrease in the thalamic perfusion is very small, or there is no change. This appears unlikely since there is no direct relationship between the magnitude of caudate decrease and thalamic increase for each Parkinsonian studied, as shown in Fig. 6.4.

Second, in all patients the 'OFF' levodopa study showed a deterioration of the perfusion of the cortex. This may have led to an increase in thalamic perfusion as a consequence of neuronal autoregulation. This would agree with the findings of Wolfson et al (1985), who reported that the rCBF in the basal ganglia contralateral to the neurological deficit in patients with unilateral Parkinson's disease was always increased with a contralateral over ipsilateral ratio of 1.14. In the same group of patients the rCMRO$_2$ showed a similar ratio of 1.12. These were significantly different from normals (1.04 and 1.05 respectively for rCBF and rCMRO$_2$). Unfortunately, no reference was made to changes observed in the thalamus. It is possible that subcortical activation may produce this thalamic effect.

A third possibility may lie in the difference in the distribution of dopamine receptors. These are different for blood vessels and for dopaminergic neurons in the basal ganglia and there are other dopamine receptors in the cortical neurons. PET studies of distribution of dopamine receptors in the human brain using 3-N-[^{11}C]methylspiperone (NMSP) showed that they are in high concentration in the head of the caudate nucleus and putamen/globus pallidus (Inoue et al 1985), with much lower concentration in the thalamus and cortex. This different receptor distribution gives different neuronal activity under the influence of levodopa which may produce different uptake and retention properties influencing the final concentration of ^{99m}Tc-HMPAO.

Conclusion

^{99m}Tc-HMPAO/SPET studies demonstrate changes in the cortical and subcortical perfusion patterns of patients with the 'ON-OFF' syndrome of Parkinson's disease. They show that levodopa induces changes of opposite direction in the head of the caudate nucleus and thalamus. Withdrawal of levodopa therapy produces a decrease in the relative concentration of the tracer in the head of the caudate nucleus and a concomitant increase in the thalamus. The effect of levodopa on blood flow may also be a consequence of activation of specific neuronal, biochemical pathways.

EPILEPSY

Epilepsy is a paroxysmal and transitory disturbance of the function of the brain which develops suddenly, ceases spontaneously, and exhibits a conspicuous tendency to recurrence (Walton 1985). In its several forms of presentation, epilepsy seems to be more a symptom than a well defined disease. The prevalence of the disease is 20/1000. In 65% of all cases there is remission for 5 years at 20-year follow up.

Aetiology

Several pathologic conditions may cause epilepsy, which gives an indication for the therapeutic approach. However the precise way in which each of these causes operates is often obscure and sometimes more than one cause can be ascribed to the clinical situation of a particular patient with epilepsy. Among the causes of epilepsy, one is considered isolated with no general basis to explain the 'fits' or 'seizures'. It is called *constitutional epilepsy* and is a confession of diagnostic failure (idiopathic epilepsy) because it simply implies that even with the most advanced methods of investigation its cause cannot be demonstrated. Treatment is always carried out with the help of anticonvulsants. However, control of epilepsy remains non-satisfactory in more than 30% of cases.

There are some patients, particularly with focal temporal lobe epilepsy which are resistant to anticonvulsant therapy and surgical treatment is considered successful (Polkey 1983). In 60 to 80% of cases with an identified focus, there is complete or near complete seizure relief after surgery although the correct side needs to be diagnosed before surgery. Patients with more than one focus are likely to continue their 'seizures' despite the removal of the temporal focus because further 'seizures' will be elicited by other focal lesions. The best surgical results are obtained in young patients in whom sclerosis in the mesial cortex of the temporal lobe is found at the operation (Falconer 1963), and in adults with attacks of hippocampal origin (Delgado-Escueta & Walsh 1985). The combination of clinical symptoms, routine EEG, and radiological studies (X-ray CT scanning) are the diagnostic aids used for the preoperative localization of epileptic foci. Good quality EEG cannot always be achieved and correct lateralization of a focus is in some situations difficult (Costa & Ell 1989a).

SPET investigations

Recently, Fish et al (1987) demonstrated the usefulness of rCBF studies with stable Xenon-enhanced CT brain scanning for the localization of foci of temporal lobe epilepsy (TLE) in patients with intractable epilepsy. An advantage of this technique is the possibility of quantification of rCBF in ml/min/100 g. In contrast, the spatial resolution with this technique is poor, mainly due to the low signal-to-noise ratio obtained in the images. Although sclerosis in the mesial cortex of the temporal lobe is the most frequent finding in patients with TLE, Fish et al (1987) reported hypoperfusion more marked in the lateral than in the mesial cortex.

^{99m}Tc-HMPAO-SPET studies cannot provide absolute values of rCBF. However, the spatial resolution is improved and relative quantitative analysis is practicable.

Patients Seven patients (5 male and 2 female) with an age range from 20 to 41 years old (average of 31.1 years) had temporal lobe epilepsy (TLE) diagnosed clinically and the foci were confirmed by ictal surface EEG. This showed that three patients had right-sided and four left-sided TLE. One patient with left TLE had a glioma in the left temporal lobe seen with the ^{99m}Tc-HMPAO-SPET, confirmed with MRI but missed by X-ray CT scanning. Another patient with left TLE had an epileptic focus in the left fronto-parietal cortex, in addition to the temporal one. Every patient underwent rCBF studies with ^{99m}Tc-HMPAO-SPET and the IGE 400AC/STARCAM and stable Xenon-enhanced CT with the IGE 9800CT/T scanner.

^{99m}Tc-HMPAO-SPET maps in patients with TLE In order to facilitate the comparison between the two rCBF tomographic techniques, slice re-orientation of the ^{99m}Tc-HMPAO-SPET data was performed to obtain brain sections through the long axis of the temporal lobe (Fig. 6.7) matching the images from the Xenon-enhanced CT study. In all studies, a non-uniform distribution of the ^{99m}Tc-HMPAO is seen. Another common feature of ^{99m}Tc-HMPAO-SPET maps of patients with epilepsy is the asymmetrical shape of the cerebrum, which may pose some orientation problems if dedicated single slice tomographs are used instead of rotating gamma cameras.

All seven patients had perfusion abnormalities detected with both rCBF techniques in the same area of the brain.

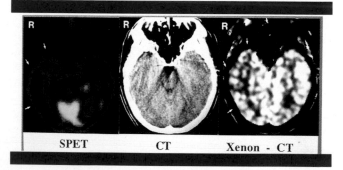

Fig. 6.7 **Comparison between ^{99m}Tc-HMPAO-SPET maps, X-ray CT and stable Xenon-enhanced CT, in a patient with right TLE.**

The Xenon-enhanced CT test always demonstrated the rCBF abnormalities confined to the lateral cortex of the temporal lobe, extending into the anterior temporal cortex, while the ^{99m}Tc-HMPAO-SPET was able to identify lesions in the mesial, lateral and anterior temporal cortex. Comparisons between the ^{99m}Tc-HMPAO-SPET data (visual and quantitative analysis) and the surface EEG findings are shown in Table 6.2.

Table 6.2 ^{99m}Tc-HMPAO-SPET findings compared to EEG in patients with epilepsy

| Patient | EEG* | Visual* | Total | Rt/Lft ratios | | |
				Ant	Mes	Lat
PMB	Rt TL	Lft TL (A+L)	1.07	1.07	1.04	1.07
DH	Lft TL	Lft TL (A+M+L)	1.06	1.14	1.24	1.17
PL	Rt TL	Rt TL (M)	0.94	–	0.92	0.96
DK	Lft TL	Lft TL (M)	1.01	–	0.93	1.01
MS	Lft TL	Lft TL (A)	0.98	0.93	1.04	0.96
KR	Rt TL	Rt TL (A+M+L)	0.87	0.88	0.93	0.92
NEC	Lft F TL	Lft F TL (L)	0.96	1.05	1.03	1.08

*Rt = right; Lft = left; F = frontal; TL = temporal lobe; A = anterior; L = lateral; M = mesial

The Rt/Lft ratios were obtained with irregular ROI delineating the whole of the temporal lobe for the values 'Total' and regular small ROI for the mesial, lateral and anterior temporal cortex. The average counts per pixel were used to calculate the ratios. These data confirm the visual localization of the perfusion abnormality in the mesial, lateral or anterior temporal cortex.

There was complete agreement between the EEG and the ^{99m}Tc-HMPAO-SPET systems but in one patient the latter localized the epileptic focus in the left temporal, opposite to the EEG findings. In this particular case (Fig. 6.7), as in all the patients studied, there was total agreement between the ^{99m}Tc-HMPAO-SPET and the Xenon-enhanced CT, in terms of lateralization. However, ^{99m}Tc-HMPAO-SPET demonstrated lesions in the mesial cortex of the temporal lobe better than did the stable Xenon-enhanced CT scanning (Compare Figs. 6.7 and 6.8).

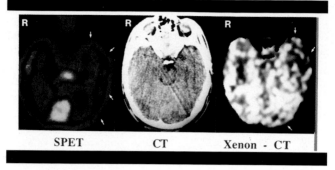

Fig. 6.8 **Comparison between** [99mTc]**-HMPAO-SPET maps, X-ray CT and stable Xenon-enhanced CT in a patient with left temporal lobe focus.**

Conclusion

[99mTc]-HMPAO-SPET studies accurately depict epileptic foci in TLE patients, during the interictal period. They entirely agree with the rCBF asymmetries found with Xenon-enhanced CT scanning.

[99mTc]-HMPAO-SPET improves the detection of perfusion abnormalities confined to the mesial and anterior cortex of the temporal lobe separated from the lateral cortical rim. In doing so it seems better than stable Xenon-enhanced CT in the evaluation of perfusion abnormalities, particularly during the pre-operative assessment of patients with TLE.

[99mTc]-HMPAO-SPET studies are also easier to perform (more widely available) and are better tolerated by patients than Xenon-CT imaging. The non-physiologic effect of the concentration of stable Xenon (needed to carry out a Xenon-CT study) on CBF should also not be minimized.

DEMENTIA

Dementia can be defined as a diffuse deterioration of the mental state due to organic (usually degenerative) disease of the brain with disorders of intellectual performance and memory as the primary clinical manifestations. It may be secondary to either intracerebral conditions (syphilis, arteriosclerosis, tumours, hydrocephalus, multiple sclerosis, virus encephalitis, etc.) or to other pathologies (eg head trauma, hypoglycaemia, neurofibromatosis, drug addiction, hypothyroidism, acquired immunodeficiency syndrome (AIDS), etc.). However, the most common forms of dementia are the senile and presenile dementias. In Britain, Rossor (1987) estimated that 1 in 14 of the 8 million men and women over the age of 65 years are demented. In Europe and USA the total number of patients with dementia is estimated at 1.5 to 2.5 millions. There are 250 000 newly-hospitalized cases per year in Europe and 470 000 in the USA.

Aetiology

Dementia of Alzheimer type (DAT) is by far the most common cause of dementia (50–60% of all cases of dementia), affecting up to 5% of the population over the age of 65 years, rising to 20% over the age of 80 years (Terry & Katzman 1983). Its aetiology is not known and treatment with the new drug tetrahydroaminoacridine (THA) is still under evaluation. In addition, 10–30% of incorrect diagnoses are made, overlooking severe depression, effect of psychopharmaceuticals, other types of dementia and mental illnesses.

There is a need for more objective studies capable of mapping out the underlying causes, mainly at the biochemical level which may contribute to a better understanding of the progression of the disease, as well as the efficacy of new developing therapies.

SPET investigations

Although ideal, receptor ligands for use with SPET to study this condition are not yet widely available. Nevertheless, ^{99m}Tc-HMPAO as a marker of brain perfusion is well suited to design a study which describes the perfusion patterns in DAT patients and follows up the natural and spontaneous progression of the disease.

Patients   Twenty DAT patients were selected from a series of consecutive referrals to the Memory Clinic at the Maudsley Hospital (Prof. Raymond Levy). Six controls were recruited from relatives of DAT patients.

All DAT patients had a standard assessment which

included clinical history, physical and mental examination, blood tests and X-ray CT scanning. The 20 DAT patients satisfied the standard criteria for the clinical diagnosis of Alzheimer's disease (McKhann et al 1984) and were subdivided into two groups according to the clinical examination:

1 Group 1 (Am) – 8 patients with amnesia as the main complaint
2 Group 2 (Ap) – 12 patients with amnesia plus aphasia and/or apraxia

Every patient underwent the following psychological tests:

1 Mini-Mental State Examination (MMSE)
2 CAMCOG battery, including among others, sections on language, memory, attention and praxis

There was no significant difference between the mean age of DAT patients (69.5 years) and the mean age of the controls (67.5 years), or between the mean age of each of the subgroups of DAT patients (72.6 years for Am; 67.4 years for Ap). There was a significant difference between these two subgroups in the psychometry performance, when testing language (Am = 26.8, Ap = 11.8; $p < 0.001$) and praxis (Am = 10.8, Ap = 5.7; $p < 0.003$). Eleven DAT patients (7 Am, 4 Ap) were followed up at the end of one year (Table 6.3).

The psychometric scores showed further deterioration of the 11 DAT patients, mainly reported to the CAMCOG examination and particularly in language performance (Table 6.4).

The two subgroups showed worsening of all the psychometric scores. However, significant differences were seen only in the CAMCOG examination scores for the Ap group and the language performance for the Am group. There was an average 16% drop in the memory scores for the Am group (4% for the Ap group) which did not reach statistical significance. Table 6.5 shows all the psychometric scores for the two subgroups of DAT patients. No DAT patient studied had any evidence of cerebral vascular disease during the period of this study.

Table 6.3 **Patients with dementia of Alzheimer type (DAT)**

	Am	Ap
n (M/F)	7 (5/2)	4 (3/1)
Age (Mean ± 1SD)	72.3 ± 11.7	67.3 ± 5.7
Age range	60 – 92	62 – 74
Follow-up time (months)	13.5 ± 1.8	13.3 ± 1.0

Table 6.4 **Psychometry of DAT patients at the time of first and repeat ^{99m}Tc-HMPAO-SPET studies**

	First	**Repeat**
MMSE	19.9 ± 4.0	16.6 ± 7.0
CAMCOG	73.1 ± 20.5	64.9 ± 23.8[b]
Language	24.0 ± 6.1	21.8 ± 7.5[a]
Memory	12.0 ± 7.6	10.5 ± 6.8
Attention	5.0 ± 2.1	4.8 ± 2.6
Praxis	9.9 ± 2.8	9.5 ± 2.7

Student's t test (paired samples): [a] – $p = 0.008$; [b] – $p = 0.01$

Brain perfusion patterns with ^{99m}Tc-HMPAO-SPET in DAT patients

A. *Visual analysis* The qualitative comparison between the pattern of brain perfusion seen with ^{99m}Tc-HMPAO and the cortical atrophy observed with X-ray CT scanning demonstrated that in the majority of the cases the perfusion abnormalities were much more extensive than the areas of cortical atrophy (Fig. 6.9) seen with the X-ray methodology.

Perfusion deficits were observed in the mesial cortex of the temporal lobes in the Am group of patients, extending, in some of them, into the lateral cortex of the temporal lobe and into the posterior parietal cortex (Fig. 6.10). In the Ap group the abnormalities were more extensive, varied from patient to patient, and included always the whole of the temporal lobe, the posterior parietal and the frontal cortex (Fig. 6.11). Although bilateral, the simple visual evaluation of the perfusion maps showed that impairment is not always symmetrical.

All the controls showed a normal brain perfusion pattern for their age. However, in the older individuals qualitative

Table 6.5 **Psychometric scores obtained by DAT patients classified in the two groups under study**

	Am		Ap	
	First	Repeat	First	Repeat
MMSE	21.9	19.1	16.5	12.0
	(2.0)	(4.9)	(4.5)	(8.5)
CAMCOG	81.3	75.0	58.8	47.3[a]
	(14.5)	(14.0)	(23.5)	(29.0)
Language	26.7	24.7[a]	19.3	16.8
	(2.0)	(3.1)	(8.4)	(10.8)
Memory	14.4	12.1	7.8	7.5
	(7.1)	(6.4)	(7.3)	(7.2)
Attention	5.9	6.0	3.5	2.8
	(0.9)	(1.2)	(2.9)	(3.4)
Praxis	10.9	10.7	8.3	7.3
	(1.9)	(1.4)	(3.6)	(3.1)

Student's t test (paired samples): [a] − $p < 0.05$ (First vs. Repeat)

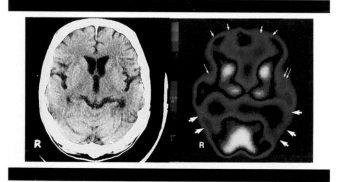

Fig. 6.9 **Comparison between ^{99m}Tc-HMPAO-SPET and X-ray CT in a patient with DAT. There is a marked difference between the degree of perfusion deficits in the frontal, temporal and posterior parietal cortex, when compared with the small degree of cortical atrophy identified with the X-ray CT on the left.**

analysis alone was insufficient to distinguish between a normal reduction in the brain perfusion related to age and one caused by underlying pathology. This was particularly noted in the analysis of transverse slices. Careful analysis

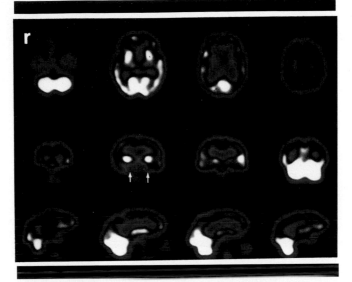

Fig. 6.10 **Perfusion deficits in a patient with DAT with amnesia as the main complaint (Am group). Only the coronal slices (middle row) display well the perfusion deficiency in the mesial cortex of both temporal lobes (small arrows), more marked on the right.**

of coronal slices helped to differentiate between normal controls and DAT subjects, which was confirmed by the quantitative analysis using cerebrum/cerebellum activity ratios. Coronal slices were always extremely valuable to study the perfusion pattern in the temporal lobes and in the superior and medial areas of the parietal lobes. In addition they enabled a clear separation between the temporal and the parietal lobes which was, at least, difficult with transverse sections.

A follow-up ^{99m}Tc-HMPAO-SPET study demonstrated further impairment of the perfusion patterns in all the cortical regions described above for the two groups of DAT patients. Interestingly, one DAT patient was investigated after being treated with THA for a very short period. However, when he was studied the drug had already been discontinued and he received no further treatment. His repeat ^{99m}Tc-HMPAO-SPET study showed some slight

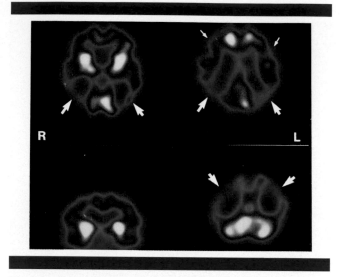

Fig. 6.11 99mTc-HMPAO-SPET maps characteristic of a patient with advanced DAT (Ap group). Arrows point to the areas of severe bilateral reduction of cortical perfusion in the posterior frontal, high and posterior parietal and temporal lobes.

improvement of the perfusion to the temporal and parietal cortex corresponding to some improvement on his psychometric scoring.

B. *Quantitative analysis* Cerebrum/cerebellum activity ratios, as described in the section on data analysis (Method III) were used to compare DAT patients with controls, as well as to determine the differences between the two groups of patients in the first and repeat studies. This quantitative analysis, carried out on coronal slices, entirely confirmed the findings of the visual analysis.

In the first study, DAT patients showed significantly lower perfusion ratios in the mesial and lateral cortex of the temporal lobes and in the posterior parietal cortex, on both hemispheres, compared to normal controls (Costa et al 1988b, Burns et al 1989). However, there were significant differences between the two groups of DAT patients; these are compared to the control values (Table 6.6).

Table 6.6 **Cerebrum/cerebellum ratios from DAT patients compared with age-matched controls**

| | | DAT | |
	Control	Am	Ap
Rt. Frontal	0.78 (0.03)	0.79 (0.02)	0.76 (0.05)
Lft. Frontal	0.79 (0.03)	0.79 (0.04)	0.75 (0.05)*
Rt. Parietal	0.79 (0.04)	0.78 (0.03)	0.77 (0.05)
Lft. Parietal	0.79 (0.04)	0.78 (0.04)	0.75 (0.05)
Rt. Lat. Temp.	0.79 (0.04)	0.75 (0.05)**	0.71 (0.04)*
Rt. Mes. Temp.	0.77 (0.04)	0.70 (0.04)	0.69 (0.04)*
Lft. Mes. Temp.	0.76 (0.03)	0.68 (0.07)	0.64 (0.07)*
Lft. Lat. Temp.	0.79 (0.04)	0.76 (0.05)**	0.66 (0.07)*
Rt. Post. Par.	0.80 (0.04)	0.77 (0.05)**	0.69 (0.09)*
Lft. Post. Par.	0.81 (0.03)	0.78 (0.04)**	0.66 (0.07)*

Student's t test (non-paired samples): $p < 0.05$ *(vs. controls); **(Am vs. Ap)

The Am group showed a statistically significant drop in the perfusion ratios for the mesial cortex of the temporal lobes. The small differences encountered in the lateral cortex of the temporal lobes and the posterior parietal cortex were not statistically significant.

In the Ap group the perfusion ratios in the whole of the temporal lobes (mesial and lateral cortex), the posterior parietal and the left frontal cortex were significantly lower than the controls, confirming the findings of the visual analysis.

This quantitative analysis confirmed that the Ap group was distinct from the Am group. The perfusion ratios in the lateral cortex of temporal lobes and posterior parietal cortex were significantly lower in the Ap group of patients.

One year follow-up The 11 DAT patients who underwent follow-up studies at one year demonstrated further impairment of the perfusion ratios in the frontal and parietal cortex of both hemispheres, as well as in the left posterior parietal (Table 6.7).

There was no difference between the cerebrum/cerebellum ratios calculated for the mesial and lateral cortex of

Table 6.7 **Perfusion ratios found in DAT patients at one year follow-up**

	First	Repeat
R/L Cerebellum	1.01 ± 0.02	1.01 ± 0.03
Rt. Lat. Temporal	0.75 ± 0.04	0.73 ± 0.02
Rt. Mes. Temporal	0.70 ± 0.03	0.70 ± 0.05
Lft. Mes. Temporal	0.67 ± 0.07	0.69 ± 0.05
Lft. Lat. Temporal	0.74 ± 0.06	0.72 ± 0.05
Rt. Frontal	0.78 ± 0.02	0.74 ± 0.02[a]
Lft. Frontal	0.78 ± 0.04	0.73 ± 0.03[a]
Rt. Parietal	0.77 ± 0.04	0.71 ± 0.04[b]
Lft. Parietal	0.76 ± 0.05	0.71 ± 0.03[c]
Rt. Post. Parietal	0.73 ± 0.10	0.71 ± 0.07
Lft. Post. Parietal	0.73 ± 0.09	0.69 ± 0.07[d]

Student's t test (paired samples): [a] – $p < 0.001$; [b] – $p = 0.002$; [c] – $p = 0.004$; [d] – $p = 0.012$

the temporal lobes. The small drop in the perfusion ratio in the right parietal cortex was not statistically significant. In addition, there was no change in the relative perfusion of the cerebellar hemispheres, which indicates that during the period of study, no patient suffered any major cerebrovascular accident. Furthermore, this was ruled out with X-ray CT scanning. Table 6.8 shows the results for the two groups of DAT patients.

The Am group had further deterioration of the perfusion ratios in the frontal, parietal and posterior parietal cortex of both hemispheres, without significant change in the temporal lobes. The Ap group showed worsening of the perfusion only in the frontal lobes, without any significant change in the rest of the cerebral cortex.

These data add an important and objective parameter to the evaluation of DAT patients. They indicate that perfusion deficits are demonstrated in patients with dementia of Alzheimer type, confined to the temporal lobes (mainly mesial cortex) in the early stages of the disease (Fig. 6.12). Later, as the disease progresses, the perfusion abnormalities extend into the posterior parietal cortex and finally into the frontal cortex (Fig. 6.13).

Table 6.8 **Perfusion ratios obtained from the two groups of DAT patients (one year follow-up)**

	Am		Ap	
	First	Repeat	First	Repeat
R/L Cerebellum	1.00	1.02	1.01	1.01
	(0.02)	(0.03)	(0.02)	(0.02)
Rt. Lat. Temporal	0.76	0.73	0.72	0.72
	(0.03)	(0.02)	(0.02)	(0.02)
Rt. Mes. Temporal	0.70	0.70	0.70	0.70
	(0.03)	(0.04)	(0.03)	(0.06)
Lft. Mes. Temporal	0.67	0.70	0.68	0.67
	(0.08)	(0.05)	(0.06)	(0.05)
Lft. Lat. Temporal	0.75	0.73	0.71	0.71
	(0.05)	(0.04)	(0.08)	(0.07)
Rt. Frontal	0.79	0.74[b]	0.78	0.74[f]
	(0.02)	(0.02)	(0.01)	(0.01)
Lft. Frontal	0.78	0.73[a]	0.78	0.73[e]
	(0.04)	(0.03)	(0.04)	(0.04)
Rt. Parietal	0.78	0.70[a]	0.74	0.72
	(0.04)	(0.01)	(0.05)	(0.07)
Lft. Parietal	0.77	0.71[d]	0.74	0.72
	(0.04)	(0.02)	(0.06)	(0.04)
Rt. Post Parietal	0.77	0.73[e]	0.66	0.67
	(0.03)	(0.04)	(0.13)	(0.11)
Lft. Post Parietal	0.77	0.71[c]	0.66	0.65
	(0.04)	(0.05)	(0.10)	(0.09)

Student's t test (paired samples): [a] $- p < 0.001$; [b] $- p = 0.002$;
[c] $- p = 0.003$; [d] $- p = 0.004$; [e] $- p = 0.008$; [f] $- p < 0.05$

Conclusion

The investigation of DAT is improved with an objective assessment of the perfusion patterns of the cerebral cortex. Cerebrum/cerebellum activity ratios of the distribution of ^{99m}Tc-HMPAO demonstrate bilateral cortical perfusion deficits, symmetrical or asymmetrical, in the temporal, posterior parietal and, later in the disease, frontal lobes. These perfusion abnormalities correlate well with the clinical assessment, particularly with the psychometric testing of intellectual performance, including among others, memory, language, attention and praxis.

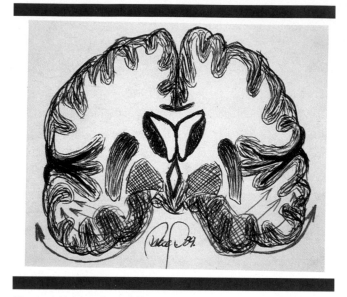

Fig. 6.12 **Progression of disease in DAT patients (1). It appears that the disease starts in the mesial cortex of the temporal lobes (red area), extending soon into the lateral cortex (red arrows).**

It is apparent from ^{99m}Tc-HMPAO-SPET studies that perfusion abnormalities commence in the temporal lobes (mesial cortex) in the early stages of the disease and extend further into the posterior parietal and frontal lobes by the late stages of advanced Alzheimer's disease.

Other types of dementia

^{99m}Tc-HMPAO-SPET studies have demonstrated cortical perfusion abnormalities in patients with non-Alzheimer frontal lobe type of dementia (Pick's disease) confined to the frontal cortex. Neary et al (1987) emphasize that these investigations provide an *in vivo* and independent marker of this dementia syndrome, which is frequently difficult to differentiate from DAT. Post-mortem examinations and cerebral cortex biopsies have shown that this clinical condition has an underlying pathophysiology distinct from that of the DAT.

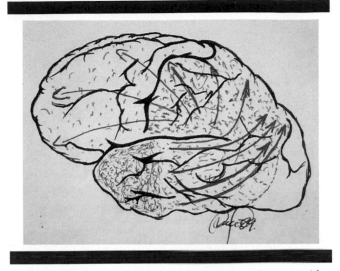

Fig. 6.13 **Progression of disease in DAT patients (as seen with** **^{99m}Tc-HMPAO-SPET) represented on a left projection of the** **brain cortex (2). From the temporal lobe the perfusion** **abnormalities extend further into the posterior parietal and, at** **late stages of the disease, into the frontal cortex.**

Multi-infarction dementia (MID) is another type of dementia (Smith et al 1988). In line with results from PET studies (Benson et al 1983), ^{99m}Tc-HMPAO-SPET studies of MID patients show abnormal perfusion patterns scattered throughout the cerebral cortex without the bilateral (symmetrical or asymmetrical) distribution patterns more typical of the DAT.

Three HIV-positive patients have been investigated with ^{99m}Tc-HMPAO-SPET. The qualitative and quantitative analysis of these patients' studies showed similar findings to DAT patients (Ell et al 1987a, Costa et al 1988b). The discrepancy between the cortical atrophy seen with X-ray CT scanning and the extent of the perfusion abnormalities observed with ^{99m}Tc-HMPAO-SPET was even more marked than that found in DAT patients, particularly group Ap (more advanced disease). Cortical perfusion deficits, with significantly reduced cerebrum/cerebellum ratios, were seen in the mesial and lateral cortex of the temporal lobes, posterior parietal, parietal and frontal cortex, similar to those found in DAT patients of group Ap.

CEREBROVASCULAR DISEASE

Cerebrovascular disease (CVD) is frequently classified in broad diagnostic categories, according to clinical criteria alone. These are, however, often inaccurate and more objective criteria are needed in order to determine prognosis, and to assess and classify populations at risk.

Aetiology

The three most common types of cerebrovascular disease are:

1 cerebral infarction
2 transient cerebral ischaemia (TIA) without infarction
3 intracranial (subarachnoid) haemorrhage

In all these types the main cause of brain (neuronal) damage is ischaemia, which may be transient (TIA) or may last for a significant length of time and therefore induce definitive brain damage (cerebral infarction/stroke). In all types of CVD significant changes in brain perfusion occur. These, as well as the consequent changes in glucose metabolism and oxygen extraction and utilization can be measured with the radioactive tracer method. PET studies have made a valuable contribution to the study of neurophysiologic and neuropathologic mechanisms in patients with cerebrovascular disease (Gibbs et al 1984). However, the development of new tracers to obtain rCBF maps with SPET broadens the applicability of these procedures to the investigation of patients with cerebrovascular disease at the District General Hospital level.

X-ray CT scanning and MRI show no abnormality in TIA. The former is often negative in acute infarction (less than 24 hours of onset), while rCBF studies offer an instantaneous assessment of the perfusion deficits characteristic of the initial stages of transient or permanent ischaemia. [99mTc]-HMPAO is the first [99mTc]-labelled radiotracer to be used with SPET for the routine assessment of CVD patients.

In general, the diagnosis of cerebral infarction is made with a clinical history in conjunction with X-ray CT scanning and MRI (these are capable of defining the type, location, and extent of the cortical and subcortical injury). Usually it is possible to distinguish a lacunar from an embolic or haemorrhagic infarction. In addition ^{99m}Tc-HMPAO-SPET will miss small size infarctions, particularly those in the white matter.

SPET investigations

What contribution can ^{99m}Tc-HMPAO-SPET make to the understanding and management of CVD?

1 ^{99m}Tc-HMPAO-SPET may play a unique role in the study of cortical changes in areas distant from the site of ischaemia, probably due to deafferentiation or diaschisis, which may be cortical (thalamic lesions) or cerebellar (large cortical infarctions)

2 ^{99m}Tc-HMPAO-SPET demonstrates cerebral infarctions immediately after the vascular insult and it may help to differentiate between TIA and infarction, particularly with follow-up studies. These will show complete recovery of the perfusion pattern after TIA, and persistent perfusion deficits during the evolution of a cerebral infarction

3 ^{99m}Tc-HMPAO-SPET shows some potential as a prognostic indicator (Costa and Ell 1989c, Launes et al 1989, Mountz et al 1990)

Patients More than 100 patients with an age range from 8 to 82 years were investigated. All the patients included were referred through the clinical routine requesting system by our colleague neurologists (stroke patients), vascular surgeons (TIA) and paediatricians (three children with systemic arterial disease, including intracranial disease). Whenever possible, X-ray CT scanning, and digital subtraction angiography were studied for comparison. Visual analysis of all the ^{99m}Tc-HMPAO-SPET studies was performed and in some particular cases quantitative analysis of the relative distribution of the tracer.

Transient ischaemic attacks (TIA)

Transient ischaemic attack (probably encompassing a heterogeneous group of patients) leads to variable changes in cerebral haemodynamics and neuronal metabolism that cannot be reliably assessed by conventional clinical and radiological criteria. The challenge in this field is to identify groups of patients at different risk and to assess responses to established or new forms of therapy.

PET studies of TIA patients between attacks have shown that a wide variety of changes in rCBF, rCBV, glucose metabolism and oxygen extraction occur in response to reduction in the cerebral perfusion pressure (CPP). Frequently, reduction in rCBF is accompanied by a relative preservation of oxygen metabolism (rCMRO$_2$), corresponding to an increase in the rOEF (regional oxygen extraction fraction) (Powers & Grubb 1987). Powers et al (1984) also showed that the greatest increase in rOEF occurred in patients with the greatest decrease in rCBF, which was indicative of greater oxygen demand at low flow rates. However, the greatest increases in rCBV were found in those patients with smallest decreases in rCBF, possibly showing that the autoregulatory capacity varied from individual to individual. Subjects with poor capacity for vasodilation would have responded with smaller increases in rCBV and greater decreases in rCBF for a given CPP. On the other hand, patients with very low CPP would have responded with lower values of rCBV and rCBF probably due to collapse of cerebral capillary vessels.

These findings demonstrate that there is little knowledge of the haemodynamics and neurophysiology of cerebral ischaemic events. As SPET is widely available, it might play an important role in the understanding of some of the mechanisms involved in the progression of cerebral ischaemia.

^{99m}Tc-HMPAO-SPET findings

All the TIA patients studied were investigated at rest between attacks. In the majority, no perfusion deficits were seen. Five patients, two of whom were studied after carotid surgery, had areas of cortical infarction clearly demonstrated by the ^{99m}Tc-HMPAO-SPET and confirmed by X-ray CT scanning.

Interesting findings were seen in a 63-year-old woman admitted with numbness and heaviness of the left arm and leg, as well as the left side of her face. This was accompanied by dysarthria. These symptoms had occurred on two previous occasions lasting for 5 minutes. In addition, she had a past history of hypothyroidism and had been on replacement therapy with thyroxine. There were no bruits in the neck. There was a >90% stenosis of the right internal carotid artery seen with DSA, and X-ray CT scanning two days after admission showed no significant abnormality. Five days after the clinical onset she underwent a 99mTc-HMPAO-SPET study which demonstrated a small area of increased tracer deposition in the right inferior parietal cortex (Fig. 6.14a). Without any further admini-

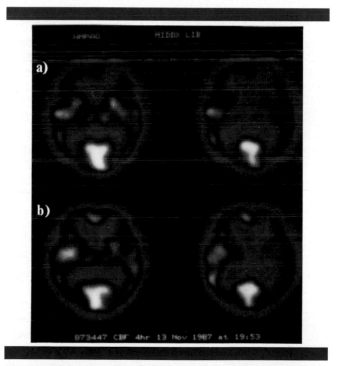

Fig. 6.14 **Clearance of 99mTc-HMPAO from an area of cerebral ischaemia in a patient with TIA. (a) – 15 minutes p.i. study; (b) – 4 hours p.i. study.**

stration of tracer, a repeat ^{99m}Tc-HMPAO-SPET was carried out 4 hours later which demonstrated reduction (15%) of tracer deposition in that area (Fig. 6.14b), probably dependent on clearance of increased blood volume at that site. Evidence that the findings of increased rCBV in areas of slight reduction of rCBF as seen by Powers et al (1985) were similarly observed with SPET, rather than PET.

One other patient, a 65-year-old woman with frequent TIAs, who had a X-ray CT scanning compatible with cerebral infarction, was studied 10 days after the acute cerebrovascular episode and showed similar ^{99m}Tc-HMPAO-SPET data. Both patients completely recovered their neurological condition during the clinical follow-up undertaken weeks later.

Cerebral infarction ('stroke')

Old infarction In well established cerebral infarction, more than one month old, a significant decrease in rCBF and $rCMRO_2$ occurs. These findings have been described by several groups who showed always a normal or slight reduction in the rOEF, suggesting a blood supply which seems to be adequate to meet the oxidative requirements of the residual tissue (Ackerman et al 1981, Lenzi et al 1982). rCBV may be either normal or decreased. It is often high relative to the rCBF values (Powers et al 1985).

Regional glucose utilization (rCMRGlu) studies in these old infarctions showed conflicting data. Some authors reported a decrease in rCMRGlu measured with ^{18}F-deoxyglucose and PET, parallel to the reduction in rCBF (Kuhl et al 1980). However, Baron et al (1983) found that the $rCMRO_2$/rCMRGlu ratio was lower in the infarcted hemisphere than in the contralateral normal, indicative of anaerobic glycolysis in the infarcted brain tissue. This anaerobic glycolysis (with very low oxygen utilization) would suggest infiltration of the infarcted area by cells other than neurons. However, the rCMRGlu method showed severe inaccuracies when applied to infarcted or even ischaemic areas, different glucose isomers showing significantly different rCMRGlu values (Gjedde et al 1985).

^{99m}Tc-HMPAO-SPET findings
What are the patterns of ^{99m}Tc-HMPAO-SPET maps in these old infarcts with reduced rCBF and rCMRO$_2$, as well as frequently reduced rCBV and rCMRGlu? All 60 patients with established infarction showed areas of severe reduction in the deposition of ^{99m}Tc-HMPAO compatible with perfusion deficits, and matching the areas of attenuation density seen on X-ray CT (Fig. 6.15), irrespective of their size (more than 2 cm) and location. Areas of infarction were found not only in the cerebral cortex, but also in deep subcortical structures. Figure 6.16 shows an example of an infarction of the right internal capsule extending into the thalamus with the corresponding X-ray CT scanning abnormality.

Crossed cerebellar diaschisis (lower tracer deposition in the contralateral cerebellar hemisphere) was always seen in large cerebral cortex infarctions (less frequently in infarctions of the occipital cortex), as well as in infarctions of subcortical structures. Due to the lower tracer uptake/

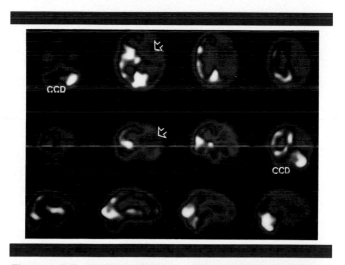

Fig. 6.15 ^{99m}Tc-HMPAO-SPET in a patient with a large cerebral infarction (arrows) in the territory of the left middle cerebral artery. Crossed cerebellar diaschisis is well demonstrated (CCD).

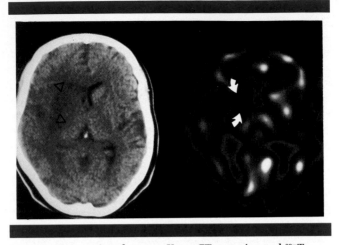

Fig. 6.16 Comparison between X-ray CT scanning and ⁹⁹ᵐTc-HMPAO-SPET in a patient with an infarction of the right internal capsule involving the ipsilateral thalamus and head of the caudate nucleus, and particularly the complex putamen/globus pallidus.

retention in the white matter, infarctions here were usually not well demonstrated unless large enough to involve adjacent grey matter structures. For instance, infarctions in the internal capsule were frequently shown by a reduction in the perfusion in the adjacent thalamus, head of the caudate nucleus and putamen/globus pallidus.

Acute and subacute stroke In acute stroke both rCBF and rCMRO$_2$ appear reduced. Wise et al (1983) reported that in half of their patients with acute stroke, there was a greater reduction in rCBF than in rCMRO$_2$, with consequent increase in oxygen extraction (rOEF). The other half had rCMRO$_2$ reduced as much as or even more than rCBF, and therefore the rOEF was normal or low. This variability in the rOEF was apparently due to individual differences in rCBF since rCMRO$_2$ varied little. The follow-up of these patients showed that in the next three to five days after the initial insult there was a further decrease in the rCMRO$_2$ while rCBF increased or decreased slightly. As a consequence, rOEF decreased, with further reduction in the rOEF during the first weeks afterwards due to an increase in rCBF and no significant change in $rCMRO_2$.

By one month, as said above, rCBF and $rCMRO_2$ were relatively matched with a normal or slightly reduced rOEF. The importance of these findings of well defined changes in rCBF and regional utilization and extraction of oxygen remains uncertain. Due to its dependency on the oxidative metabolism, the most important determinant of functional integrity of the brain appears to be the $rCMRO_2$. However, the clinical outcome appears not to correlate with an increase or decrease in the $rCMRO_2$ (Wise et al 1983).

^{99m}Tc-HMPAO-SPET findings In acute stroke, less than 24 hours after onset, ^{99m}Tc-HMPAO-SPET studies show a characteristic lack of perfusion in the arterial territory involved in the ischaemic insult, even in the absence of X-ray CT scanning changes (Fig. 6.17). In the following day, a partial recovery can be observed, particularly around the edge of the infarcted tissue. There appears to be no evidence of rebound increase in tracer deposition indicative of increased rCBF ('luxury perfusion' or 'reactive hyperaemia'). Marked increases in the ^{99m}Tc HMPAO uptake/retention were seen in several patients studied between day 6 and day 15 from clinical onset of stroke. This 'reactive hyperaemia' is often so intense that it creates difficulties for the display of the rest of the brain. Crossed cerebellar diaschisis was always demonstrated from day 1 and remained until the latest stages (15 days, 40 days and even in infarctions as old as three years).

These findings correlate with the previously described reduction in the rCBF and cerebral utilization of oxygen observed with PET studies. They are similar to the patterns described for the rCMRGlu.

Conclusion

^{99m}Tc-HMPAO-SPET contributes to the study of the neurophysiologic mechanisms underlying acute cerebral infarction, highlighting changes which occur in areas distant from the site of primary stroke (deafferentiation or diaschisis).

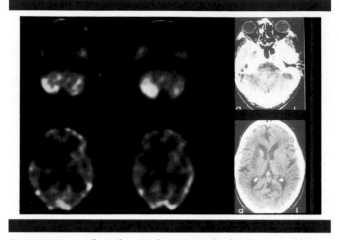

Fig. 6.17 Acute (less than 24 hours) cerebral infarction. The
99mTc-HMPAO-SPET seen on the left was undertaken 18 hours
after the clinical onset. Impaired perfusion is seen involving
the right internal capsule, the head of the caudate nucleus, the
putamen/globus pallidus and the thalamus, extending into the
temporal and parietal cortex on the same hemisphere. A repeat
study was carried out on the following day. The area of
reduced perfusion is confined to the subcortical structures with
an almost normal cortical uptake. X-ray CT scanning
performed a few hours later (right side of the figure) showed
the lesion in the projection of the internal capsule.

99mTc-HMPAO-SPET identifies acute stroke less than
12–24 hours after the clinical onset, when X-ray CT
scanning is often (particularly when non-haemorrhagic)
negative.

There is increasing evidence that 99mTc-HMPAO-SPET
studies have a possible role in the prognostic assessment
of patients with stroke.

SPACE-OCCUPYING DISEASES

An intracranial space-occupying lesion (SOL) involves any
abnormality, whether vascular, neoplastic or inflammatory
in origin, which may increase the volume of the intracranial

contents and thus lead to a rise in the intracranial pressure (Walton 1985). This definition suggests that there is always a breakdown in the BBB. The past success of the radiotracer method for the detection of these intracranial lesions was based upon the ability of ^{99m}Tc (mainly as pertechnetate) to demonstrate sites of disruption of the BBB.

With the advent of X-ray CT scanning and more recently MRI, the clinical demand for classical BBB imaging has dropped. The anatomical information required by the surgeon is electively given by X-ray CT and MR imaging. Even radiotherapy planning benefits from the spatial resolution of these two imaging modalities, which may supply an accurate measurement of the volume of the space-occupying lesion.

Nowadays more and more patients with intracranial tumours receive chemotherapy. The ultimate fate of this therapy is dependent upon the vascular supply to the tumour and its metabolic (biochemical) rate. The study of blood flow and glucose metabolism of the tumour has been recognized as important.

SPET investigations

Di Chiro (1985) showed in a review of 100 PET studies of brain tumours, using ^{18}F-2-deoxyglucose (FDG), that it was possible to discriminate the hypermetabolic neoplastic mass from the central hypometabolic area related to the post-chemotherapy necrosis. Tumour grading is an aim of the PET-FDG or even amino-acid method.

Patients Forty patients with an age range from 19 to 82 years old were studied; 11 patients were referred with probable brain metastases, but which were subsequently not confirmed either on the conventional BBB/SPET study, or the ^{99m}Tc-HMPAO-SPET. These served as controls for the definition of cortical and subcortical normal perfusion patterns.

The other 29 patients had the following diagnoses of space-occupying lesions confirmed by surgery, biopsy and other imaging modalities, including X-ray CT scanning and DSA:

Diagnosis	No. of patients
Primary tumours	
Low grade glioma	2
High grade glioma	4
Astrocytoma	1
Meningioma	2
Neuroblastoma	1
Haemangioblastoma	1
Metastases	
Ca. Breast	3
Ca. Lung	7
Others	5
AVM	3

^{99m}Tc-HMPAO-SPET findings   Three cases in this series showed intense tumour uptake of ^{99m}Tc-HMPAO, higher than cerebral and cerebellar cortex: one neuroblastoma (Fig. 6.18), one haemangioblastoma and one meningioma. In the other 27 cases of space-occupying lesions the distribution pattern of ^{99m}Tc-HMPAO was consistently lower

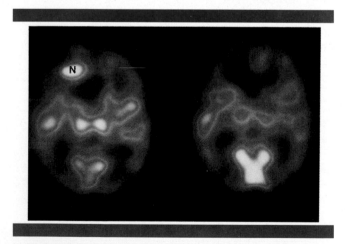

Fig. 6.18 Increased concentration of ^{99m}Tc-HMPAO in a neuroblastoma (N) of the right retro-orbital area, extending into the frontal cortex, before (left) and three months after radiotherapy (right).

than cerebral cortex (Fig. 6.19), in contrast to reports by other authors (Langen et al 1987, Flower et al 1989).

Langen et al (1987) showed that tracer uptake in high grade malignant gliomas was variable. In 8 out of 25 cases the tumour uptake was greater than the cerebral cortex uptake. It was always reduced in low grade malignant gliomas and 3 out of 5 meningiomas showed high ^{99m}Tc-HMPAO uptake. These authors also reported reduction in the tumour uptake after radiotherapy and chemotherapy. All other tumours including metastases demonstrated no uptake of ^{99m}Tc-HMPAO. Flower et al (1989) found similar variability, reporting that gliomas had increased, normal or decreased ^{99m}Tc-HMPAO uptake, while metastases showed equal or lower uptake but never higher than the cerebral cortex. After radiotherapy there was reduction in the tumour uptake (as reported by Langen et al 1987). However in six patients a significant increase (the greatest being +44%) in the uptake of ^{99m}Tc-HMPAO was found after radiotherapy. They concluded that the wide spectrum in such tumour uptake was a reflection of large variations in tumour blood flow.

Another study of ^{99m}Tc-HMPAO uptake in tumours (Lindegaard et al 1986) clearly demonstrated that, at least in two hypervascular tumours, uptake was similar to that in tumours without hypervascularity. They studied 12

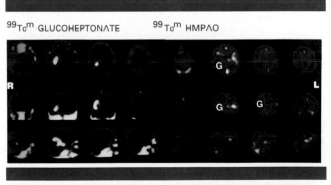

Fig. 6.19 **Comparison between classical BBB/SPET (left) and ^{99m}Tc-HMPAO-SPET (right) in a patient with malignant glioma (G).**

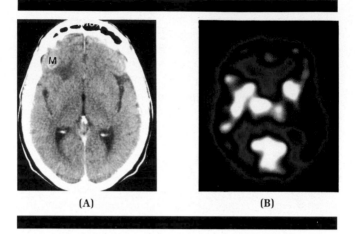

(A) (B)

Fig. 6.20 **Comparison between (A) X-ray CT scanning and (B) 99mTc-HMPAO-SPET maps in a case of single small frontal cortex metastasis.**

patients with cerebral glioma of different grades and vascularity (assessed by intra-arterial DSA) and showed in all cases significant reduction of the 99mTc-HMPAO tumour uptake.

Comparing 99mTc-HMPAO-SPET and X-ray CT scanning

Frequently the area of decreased 99mTc-HMPAO concentration is larger than the tumour itself, and this correlates well with the distribution of oedema seen with X-ray CT scanning (Ell et al 1987b). In one case of a small (2×2 cm) frontal cortex metastasis of carcinoma of the lung the 99mTc-HMPAO-SPET maps showed it less clearly than did X-ray CT scanning (Fig. 6.20).

Cerebral 'steal' in brain tissue surrounding AVMs

In two cases of cerebral cortex arteriovenous malformations (AVM), it was possible to demonstrate what has been previously described as the 'steal' phenomenon. This is produced by a shift in the perfusion rates from the cortex surrounding an AVM due to the high flow rates through the AVM itself (Feindel et al 1971). The concept behind this 'steal' is that the presence of vessels of very low resistance in the AVM produces a shunt condition which compromizes nutrient flow and perfusion to adjacent areas of the brain.

Cerebral 'steal' has been demonstrated by Lassen & Pálvölgyi (1968) who showed that an area of ischaemia due to reduced rCBF had a further reduction in blood flow in response to elevated arterial CO_2. The inverse was observed with hypocapnia. The following two case reports illustrate the cerebral 'steal' observed with ^{99m}Tc-HMPAO-SPET.

Case 1 – response to hypercapnia   A 79-year-old man with right parietal parasagittal AVM for 36 years. He suffered from recurring episodes of weakness of the left leg lasting for 10 minutes with complete recovery afterwards.

A ^{99m}Tc-HMPAO-SPET study at rest showed the lack of perfusion in the area occupied by the AVM of the right parietal cortex (Fig. 6.21A), surrounded by a strip of reasonable cortical perfusion. The patient had a repeat study one week later to investigate the response to hypercapnia. He breathed a mixture of CO_2 (6%) in air for 10 minutes and ^{99m}Tc-HMPAO was intravenously injected after 8 minutes. His blood pressure at rest equalled 130/70 mmHg, heart rate was 60 beats per minute and the end-tidal CO_2 30.0 mmHg. By the time of the injection of ^{99m}Tc-HMPAO the blood pressure was 160/90 mmHg, the heart rate 90 beats per minute and the end-tidal CO_2 51.5 mmHg. There was an increase of 72% in the end-tidal CO_2 as well as significant increments in both the blood pressure and heart rate, demonstrating good haemodynamic response to the hypercapnic stimulus.

The repeat ^{99m}Tc-HMPAO-SPET investigation demonstrated the same pattern of lack of perfusion in the area of the AVM. In addition, there was a significant reduction in the concentration of ^{99m}Tc-HMPAO in the surrounding cortex (Fig. 6.21B) compatible with impairment of regional cortical perfusion, due to the 'cerebral steal', made worse by the hypercapnic stimulus.

Case 2 – response to hypocapnia   A 26-year-old woman with a six-year history of intermittent headache with

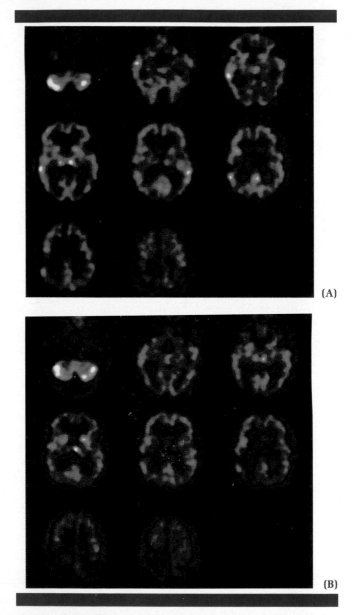

(A)

(B)

Fig. 6.21 ^{99m}Tc-HMPAO-SPET maps (A) at rest and (B) after CO_2 stimulation in an AVM of the posterior parietal cortex.

'blackouts', thought to be due to an underlying epilepsy. X-ray CT scanning and DSA showed an AVM in the left occipital lobe. The resting ⁹⁹ᵐTc-HMPAO-SPET study demonstrated the lack of perfusion in the area of the AVM with surrounding ischaemia (Fig. 6.22, upper).

The patient agreed to undergo a second ⁹⁹ᵐTc-HMPAO-SPET investigation during voluntary hyperventilation in order to achieve hypocapnia. She hyperventilated for 5 minutes and ⁹⁹ᵐTc-HMPAO was administered in an antecubital vein after 3 minutes. By 5 minutes she felt unwell without developing any seizure. The hypocapnic ⁹⁹ᵐTc-HMPAO-SPET transverse maps (Fig. 6.22, lower)

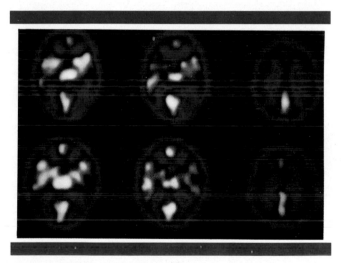

Fig. 6.22 **⁹⁹ᵐTc-HMPAO-SPET maps in a patient with an AVM of the left posterior parietal cortex, at rest (upper) and during hypocapnia (lower).**

clearly demonstrated that the area of reduction in perfusion in the occipital lobe was smaller than in the resting study. There was a well defined rim of perfused occipital cortex surrounding the AVM, compatible with the reverse of the 'cerebral steal'.

Conclusion
It appears that the ⁹⁹ᵐTc-HMPAO uptake in tumours is not

only dependent on the blood flow to the tumour but may also be influenced by its metabolic rate. In support of this contention is the fact that tumours composed of young (probably with low differentiation) cells and relatively high metabolic rates, such as haemangioblastoma and neuroblastoma show intense tracer concentration. In addition, tumours with different vascularity may show similar ^{99m}Tc-HMPAO uptake patterns and tumours of similar histology may evolve in a rather dissimilar manner (Walter 1985). It is therefore not surprising that the distribution of the blood flow-mediated tracer in tumours will not always be identical. Findings by Flower et al (1989) suggest that the higher the ^{99m}Tc-HMPAO uptake in the tumour the better the response to therapy. Whether this demonstrates a blood flow effect or a consequence of differing radiosensitivities, is still unclear.

REFERENCES

Ackerman RH, Correia JA, Alpert NM, et al 1981 Positron imaging in ischaemic stroke disease using compounds labelled with oxygen-15. Archives of Neurology **38**: 537–543

Andersen AR, Friberg L, Olesen TS, Olesen J 1988 Delayed hyperemia following hypoperfusion in classical migraine. Single photon emission computed tomographic demonstration. Archives of Neurology **45**: 154–159

Baron JC, Rougemont D, Soussaline F, Crouzel C, Bousser MG, Comar D 1983 Positron tomography investigation of local coupling among CBF, oxygen consumption, and glucose utilization. Journal of Cerebral Blood Flow Metabolism **3**: S242–S243

Benson DF, Kuhl DE, Hawkins RA, Phelps ME, Cummings JL, Tsai SY 1983 The fluorodeoxyglucose ^{18}F scan in Alzheimer's disease and multi-infarct dementia. Archives of Neurology **40**: 711–714

Burns A, Philpot M, Costa DC, Ell PJ, Levy R 1989 The investigation of Alzheimer's disease with single photon emission tomography. Journal of Neurology, Neurosurgery, and Psychiatry **52**: 248–253

Costa DC, Burns A, Philpot M, Ell PJ, Levy R 1989b One year follow-up of dementia of Alzheimer type (DAT) patients:

clinical and rCBF/SPET correlations. Nuclear Medicine Communications **10**: 232

Costa DC, Davies PTG, Jones BE, Steiner TJ, Jewkes RF, Clifford Rose F 1988a ⁹⁹ᵐTc-HMPAO studies in patients with migraine, tension and cluster headache. Nuclear Medicine Communications **9**: 196–197

Costa DC, Ell PJ 1989a Focal temporal lobe epilepsy; oblique reconstruction and slice re-orientation improves HMPAO/SPET analysis. Nuclear Medicine Communications **10**: 231

Costa DC, Ell PJ 1989c ⁹⁹ᵐTc-HMPAO Washout in Prognosis of Stroke. The Lancet **i**: 213–214

Costa DC, Ell PJ, Burns A, Philpot M, Levy R 1988b CBF Tomograms with ⁹⁹ᵐTc-HMPAO in patients with dementia (Alzheimer type and HIV) and Parkinson's disease – initial results. Journal of Cerebral Blood Flow and Metabolism **8**: S109–S115

Delgado-Escueta AV, Walsh GO 1985 Type 1 complex seizures of hippocampal origin: excellent results of anterior temporal lobectomy. Neurology **35**: 143–154

Di Chiro G 1985 Brain imaging of glucose utilisation in cerebral tumours. In: Sokoloff L (ed) Brain Imaging and Brain Function. Association for Research in Nervous and Mental Disease. Raven Press, New York, **63**: pp. 185–197

Ell PJ, Costa DC, Harrison MGJ 1987a Imaging cerebral damage in HIV infection. The Lancet **ii**: 569–570

Ell PJ, Jarritt PH, Costa DC, Cullum ID, Lui D 1987b Functional imaging of the brain. Seminars in Nuclear Medicine **17**: 214–229

Falconer MA, Serafetinides EA 1963 A follow up study of surgery in temporal lobe epilepsy. Journal of Neurology, Neurosurgery and Psychiatry **26**: 154–165

Feindel W, Yamamota YL, Hodge CP 1971 Red cerebral veins and the cerebral steal syndrome: Evidence from fluoroscein angiography and microregional blood flow by radioisotopes during excision of an angioma. Journal of Neurosurgery **35**: 167–179

Fish DR, Lewis TT, Brooks DJ, Zilkha E, Wise RJS, Kendall BE 1987 Regional cerebral blood flow of patients with focal epilepsy studied using xenon enhanced CT brain scanning. Journal of Neurology, Neurosurgery and Psychiatry **50**: 1584–1588

Flower MA, Babich JW, Keeling F et al 1989 Clinical evaluation of a new radioactive tracer ^{99m}Tc-HMPAO for imaging regional cerebral blood flow in patients with brain tumours. In: Angerson WJ, Sheldon CD, Barbenel JC, Fisher AC, Gaylor JDS (eds). Blood Flow In The Brain, Clarendon Press, Oxford, pp. 50–59

Gibbs JM, Wise RJS, Leenders KL, Jones T 1984 Evaluation of cerebral perfusion reserve in patients with carotid artery occlusion. The Lancet i: 310–314

Gjedde A, Weinhard K, Heiss W-D et al 1985 Comparative regional analysis of 2-fluorodeoxyglucose and methyl glucose uptake in brain of four stroke patients with special reference to the regional estimation of the lumped constant. Journal of Cerebral Blood Flow and Metabolism 5: 163–178

Hornykiewicz O 1972 Neurochemistry of Parkinsonism. In Lajtha A (ed). Handbook of Neurochemistry, Plenum Press, New York, pp. 465–501

Inoue Y, Wagner HN, Wong DF et al 1985 Atlas of dopamine receptor images (PET) of the human brain. Journal of Computer Assisted Tomography 9: 129–140

Kuhl DE, Phelps ME, Kowell AP, Metter EJ, Selin C, Winter J 1980 Effects of stroke on local cerebral metabolism and perfusion: mapping by emission computed tomography of ^{18}FDG and ^{13}NH$_3$. Annals of Neurology 8: 47–60

Langen K-J, Roosen N, Kuwert T et al 1987 ^{99m}Tc-HMPAO-SPET in the study of cerebral tumours: results in 40 patients. Nuclear Medicine 26: 118

Lassen NA, Pálvölgyi R 1968 Cerebral steal during hypercapnia observed by the 133-xenon technique in man. Scandinavian Journal of Clinical Laboratory Investigations 22 (Suppl. 102) XIII: D

Launes J, Nikkinan P, Lindroth L, Brownell AL, Liewendahl K, Livanainen M 1989 Brain perfusion defect size in SPET predicts outcome in cerebral infarction. Nuclear Medicine Communications 10: 981–990

Lauritzen M, Olesen J 1984 Regional cerebral blood flow during migraine attacks by Xenon-133 inhalation and emission tomography. Brain 107: 447–461

Leão AAP 1944 Spreading depression of activity in cerebral cortex. Journal of Neurophysiology 7: 359–390

Leenders KL, Wolfson L, Gibbs JM, Wise RJS, Causon R, Jones

T, Legg NJ 1985 The effect of L-dopa on regional cerebral blood flow and oxygen metabolism in patients with Parkinson's disease. Brain 108: 171–191

Lenzi GL, Frackowiak RSJ, Jones T 1982 Cerebral oxygen metabolism and blood flow in human cerebral ischaemic infarction. Journal of Cerebral Blood Flow and Metabolism 2: 321–335

Levine SR, Welch KMA, Ewing JR, Joseph R 1987 Cerebral blood flow asymmetries in migraine. In: Rose FC (ed). Current Problems in Neurology: 4 Advances in Headache Research. John Libbey & Company Ltd, London, pp. 71–74

Lindegaard MW, Skretting A, Hager B, Watne K, Lindegaard K-F 1986 Cerebral and cerebellar uptake of $^{99m}Tc(d,l)$-hexamethyl-propylene amine oxime (HMPAO) in patients with brain tumour studied by single photon emission computerized tomography. European Journal of Nuclear Medicine 12: 417–420

Marsden CD, Parkes JD 1976 'On-Off' effects in patients with Parkinson's disease on chronic levodopa therapy. The Lancet i: 292–296

McKhann G, Drachman D, Folstein M, Katzman R, Price D, Stadlan EM 1984 Clinical diagnosis of Alzheimer's disease: report of the NINCDS-ADRDA work group under the auspices of the Department of Health and Human Services Task Force in Alzheimer's Disease. Neurology 34: 939–944

Mountz JM, Modell JG, Foster NL et al 1990 Prognostication of recovery following stroke using the comparison of CT and Technetium-^{99m}Tc-HMPAO-SPET. Journal of Nuclear Medicine 31: 61-66

Muenter MM, Tyce GM 1971 L-dopa therapy of Parkinson's disease: plasma L-dopa concentration, therapeutic response, and side effects. Mayo Clinic Proceedings 46: 231–239

Neary D, Snowden JS, Shields RA et al 1987 Single photon emission tomography using ^{99m}Tc-HMPAO in the investigation of dementia. Journal of Neurology, Neurosurgery and Psychiatry 50: 1101–1109

Nutt JG, Woodward WR, Hammerstad JP, Carter JH, Andersen JL 1984 The 'ON-OFF' phenomenon in Parkinson's disease. Relation to levodopa absorption and transport. New England Journal of Medicine 310 (8): 483–488

Olesen J, Larsen B, Lauritzen M 1981a Focal hyperemia

followed by spreading oligemia and impaired activation of rCBF in classical migraine. Annals of Neurology **9**: 344–352

Olesen J, Tfelt-Hansen P, Henriksen L, Larsen B 1981b The common migraine attack may not be initiated by cerebral ischaemia. The Lancet **ii**: 438–440

Polkey CE 1983 Effects of anterior temporal lobectomy apart from the relief of seizures: a study of 40 patients. Journal of the Royal Society of Medicine **76**: 354–358

Powers WJ, Grubb RL Jr 1987 Hemodynamic and metabolic relationships in cerebral ischaemia and subarachnoid haemorrhage. In: Wood JH (ed) Cerebral Blood Flow – Physiological and Clinical Aspects. McGraw-Hill, New York, pp. 387–401

Powers WJ, Grubb RL Jr, Raichle ME 1984 Physiological responses to focal cerebral ischaemia in humans. Annals of Neurology **16**: 546–552

Powers WJ, Raichle ME, Grubb RL Jr 1985 Positron emission tomography to assess cerebral perfusion. The Lancet **i**: 102–103

Rossor MN 1987 Dementia. British Journal of Hospital Medicine **38**: 47–50

Smith FW, Besson JAO, Gemmell HG, Sharp PF 1988 The use of Technetium-99m-HMPAO in the assessment of patients with dementia and other neuropsychiatric conditions. Journal of Cerebral Blood Flow and Metabolism **8**: S116–S122

Terry RD, Katzman R 1983 Senile dementia of Alzheimer type. Annals of Neurology **14**: 497–506

Uhl GR, Hedreen JC, Price DL 1985 Parkinson's disease: loss of neurons from the ventral tegmental area contralateral to therapeutic surgical lesions. Neurology **35**: 1215–1218

Vahlquist B 1955 Migraine in children. International Archives of Allergy and Applied Immunology **7**: 348–355

Walton Sir J 1985 Brain's disease of the nervous system (Ninth ed) Oxford University Press, Oxford

Warner C, Brown LL, Wolfson LI 1982 L-dopa produces regional changes in glucose utilisation which form discrete anatomic patterns in motor nuclei and hypothalamus of rats. Experimental Neurology **78**: 591–601

CASE 1

A 2-year-old girl with recurrent grand mal seizures and episodes of alternating hemiparesis had multiple areas of infarction on computed tomography (Fig. 7.1). Magnetic resonance imaging showed cortical atrophy particularly in the right frontal, sylvian, and occipital regions (Fig. 7.2). Both middle cerebral arteries were virtually occluded, and Moya moya vessels in the region of the striate perforators were seen on angiography (Fig. 7.3). Transcranial Doppler failed to identify the middle cerebral arteries and showed elevated vertebrobasilar velocities (Fig. 7.4) suggesting collateral posterior circulation supply.

Cerebral blood flow, as demonstrated by SPET, was grossly abnormal with multiple bilateral areas of hypoperfusion (Fig. 7.5, upper and Fig. 7.6, upper) and an area of hyperperfusion in the left frontal and left fronto-

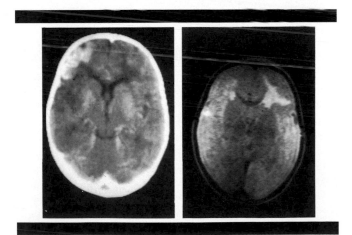

Fig. 7.1   Fig. 7.2

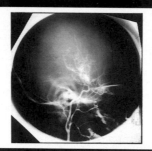

Fig. 7.3

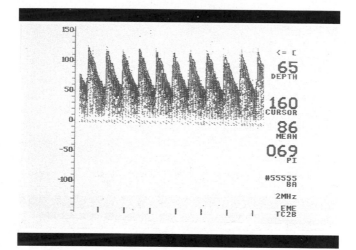

Fig. 7.4

parietal region (Fig. 7.6, upper). Bilateral encephalo-duro-arterio-synangiosis was performed in an attempt to improve cerebral perfusion. Despite this, further ischaemic damage was evident on MRI scanning six months post-operatively (Fig. 7.7). Repeat SPET scanning (Fig. 7.5, lower and Fig. 7.6, lower) showed more widespread hypoperfusion also involving the previous area of hyperperfusion, apparently indicating an area of luxury perfusion on the initial scan.

The case shows the value of SPET in following progress after neurovascular surgery.

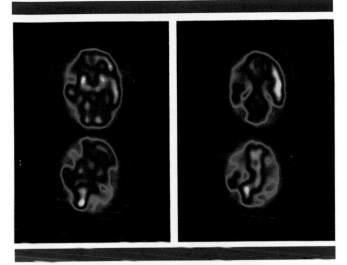

Fig. 7.5   Fig. 7.6

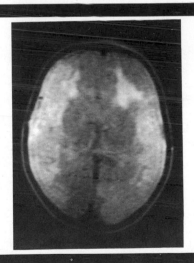

Fig. 7.7

CASE 2

A 25-year-old man with sudden onset of headache was shown to have subarachnoid haemorrhage with a right sylvian haematoma (Fig. 7.8). Angiography showed a right middle cerebral aneurysm, and there was spasm of the right internal carotid artery and the proximal segments of

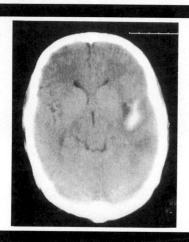

Fig. 7.8

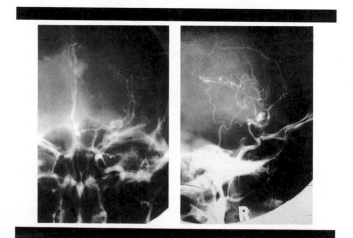

Fig. 7.9   Fig. 7.10

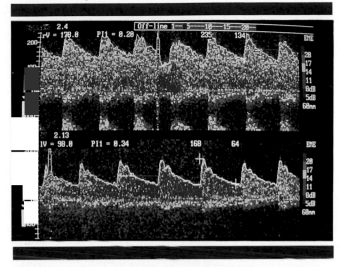

Fig. 7.11

the right middle and anterior cerebral arteries (Figs. 7.9, 7.10). Transcranial Doppler velocities were raised at the time of angiography, and increased even further, consistent with worsening vasospasm (Fig. 7.11). The patient then developed a dense left hemiparesis.

SPET showed an area of hypoperfusion surrounded by intense hyperperfusion (Fig. 7.12 and Fig. 7.13, upper). Repeat SPET two weeks later showed hypoperfusion at the site of permanent ischaemic damage, with disappearance

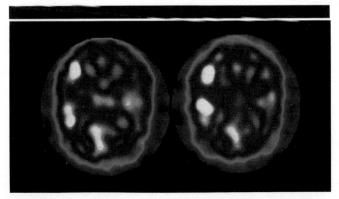

Fig. 7.12

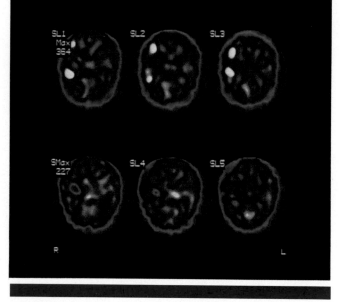

Fig. 7.13

of the intensely perfused areas (Fig. 7.13, lower and Fig. 7.14).

The case illustrates the appearance on SPET scanning in patients who have recently developed delayed ischaemic deficit after subarachnoid haemorrhage.

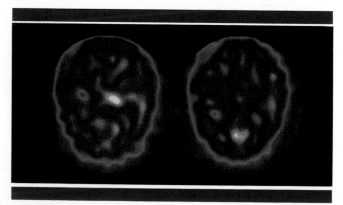

Fig. 7.14

CASE 3

A 55-year-old woman with a subarachnoid haemorrhage (Fig. 7.15) from a ruptured left internal carotid artery (Fig. 7.16), was well on admission (WFNS Grade 1). She became increasingly drowsy, and this was accompanied by an increase in Doppler flow velocities on the left anterior and middle cerebral arteries.

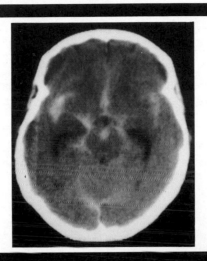

Fig. 7.15

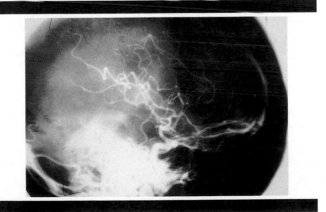

Fig. 7.16

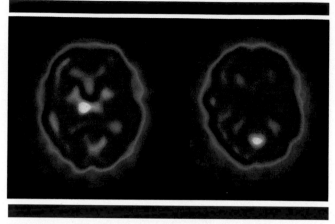

Fig. 7.17

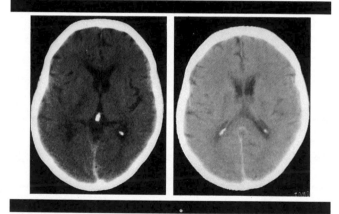

Fig. 7.18   Fig. 7.19

SPET showed left hemisphere hypoperfusion (Fig. 7.17). Right hemiparesis ensued the following day, and CT scanning suggested left basal ganglia infarction (Fig. 7.18), which was more clearly seen on repeat CT one week later (Fig. 7.19).

The case illustrates the value of SPET scanning in the early detection of focal perfusion defects due to delayed vasospasm after subarachnoid haemorrhage.

CASE 4

A 29-year-old woman with three weeks of constant right-sided headache was found to have a systolic bruit on the right side of the neck and cranium. CT scan was normal (Fig. 7.20). Transcranial Doppler (TCD) showed very high right internal carotid artery velocities (Fig. 7.21). Angiography showed a right carotid-cavernous fistula, and fibromuscular dysplasia of carotid and vertebral arteries. MRI showed the fistula and dilated superior ophthalmic veins, especially on the right (Fig. 7.22). Collateral right hemisphere circulation was assessed prior to balloon embolization of the fistula, as this procedure necessitated occlusion of the right internal carotid artery.

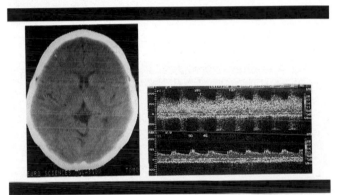

Fig. 7.20   Fig. 7.21

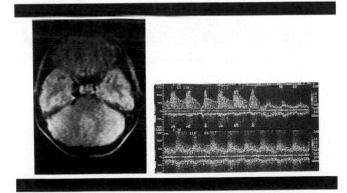

Fig. 7.22   Fig. 7.23

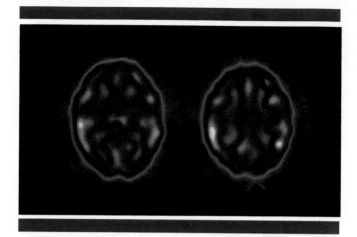

Fig. 7.24

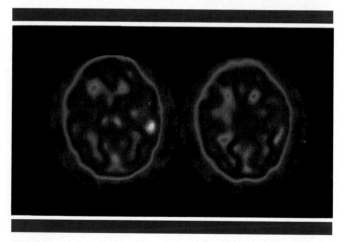

Fig. 7.25

During test carotid compression, middle cerebral artery velocity dropped (Fig. 7.23, upper) but returned to baseline after 20 seconds (Fig. 7.23, lower). Resting SPET scan was normal (Fig. 7.24), but during carotid compression showed right-sided hypoperfusion with hemisphere asymmetry of 20% (Fig. 7.25).

After balloon insertion (Figs. 7.26, 7.27), repeat MRI

showed no ischaemic change (Fig. 7.28), and repeat SPET
showed symmetrical perfusion (Fig. 7.29).

The case illustrates that collateral flow may compensate
a hemisphere perfusion asymmetry of 20%, as assessed by
SPET, after carotid occlusion.

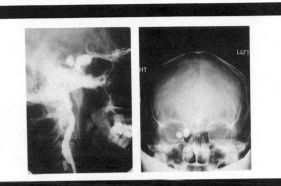

Fig. 7.26   *Fig. 7.27*

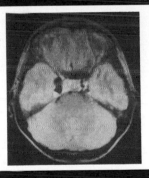

Fig. 7.28

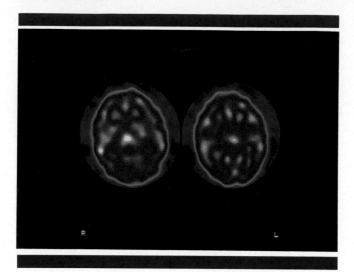

Fig. 7.29

CASE 5

A 48-year-old woman with Takayasu's arteritis was investigated for attacks of light-headedness and vertigo. Right carotid and arm pulses were absent and there was a bruit over the left carotid artery. Arch aortography showed innominate occlusion and left subclavian stenosis (Fig. 7.30). CT scan was normal. Transcranial Doppler showed increased velocity in the left anterior cerebral artery (ACA), reversed and turbulent flow in the right ACA, and a left-to-right vertebrovertebral shunt (Fig. 7.31); velocities in the right middle cerebral artery were reduced compared to the left.

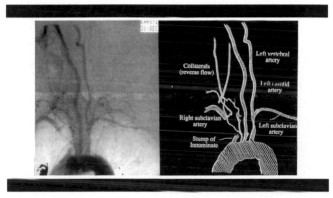

Fig. 7.30

These findings suggested that the most vulnerable area of the cerebral circulation was in the right hemisphere, in the watershed between the two remaining major cerebral supply vessels, namely the left carotid and left vertebral arteries. This area was identified on SPET scanning: an area of hypoperfusion in the right anterior hemisphere (Figs. 7.32, 7.33).

The case shows the use of SPET in defining regional perfusion patterns in cases of proximal arterial disease in the cerebral supply vessels.

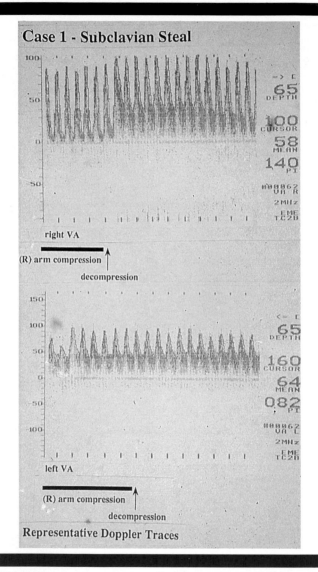

Fig. 7.31

122

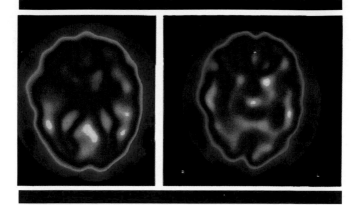

Fig. 7.32   Fig. 7.33

CASE 6

An 8-year-old girl with sudden onset hemiparesis, left homonymous hemianopia, and left seventh and twelfth cranial nerve palsy, had a right middle cerebral artery territory infarct (Figs. 7.34, 7.35). Cerebral angiography showed a focal stenotic lesion on the right middle cerebral artery, and a intimal flap in distal internal carotid and proximal middle cerebral arteries (Fig. 7.36). Transcranial Doppler showed increased velocities over the stenotic segment, with marked slowing distally (Figs. 7.37, 7.38);

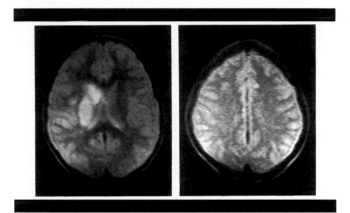

Fig. 7.34   Fig. 7.35

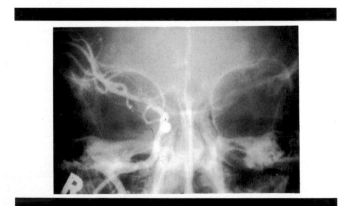

Fig. 7.36

Fig. 7.37

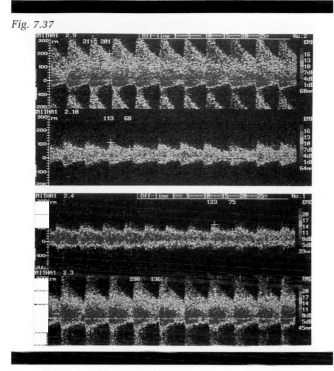

Fig. 7.38

and there was increased basilar artery velocity suggesting collateral flow from the posterior circulation.

SPET showed reduced flow in the entire right hemisphere (Figs. 7.39, 7.40).

Follow up of this case, using SPET and Doppler, will assess patterns of cerebral perfusion, and determine the need for microvascular cerebral revascularization.

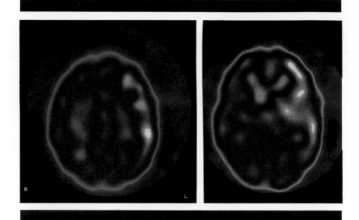

Fig. 7.39   Fig. 7.40

CASE 7

A 32-year-old woman with a history of epilepsy since the age of 5. Her seizures were mostly partial but occasionally became generalized. The partial seizures involved a variety of manifestations. She had occasional twilight states which appeared to be ictal, whereby she was only partially responsive, could move around and co-operate to a limited extent, but was considerably cognitively impaired. Her frank complex partial seizures were preceded by an aura which she was unable to describe. She would then have a stare and may have had twitching on the right side of her mouth. These attacks tended to come in runs. Despite

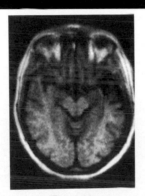

Fig. 7.41

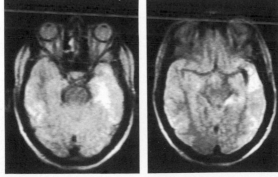

Fig. 7.42   *Fig. 7.43*

maximal anti-convulsant therapy she never had anything than poor seizure control. Seizure frequency was up to 12 per day, and she suffered progressive cognitive impairment mainly relating to the function of the left temporal lobe.

Many ictal EEG recordings showed seizure onset in the left temporal lobe; foramen ovale recordings showed a left mesial origin for the seizures. The T1 weighted MRI scan (Fig. 7.41) showed atrophy of the medial aspect of the left temporal lobe which was characterized by an increased T2 signal in the adjacent white and grey matter on the T2 weighted scans (Figs. 7.42, 7.43).

Interictal SPET scanning (Fig. 7.44, upper) demonstrated marked hypoperfusion of the whole of the left temporal lobe. Similar appearances were found in a scan carried out 50 seconds after a seizure (Fig. 7.44, lower). In contrast, SPET carried out during one of her twilight states (Fig. 7.45, upper) showed a marked increase in signal in the mesial aspect of the left temporal lobe, in an area

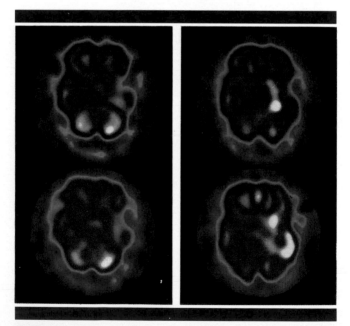

Fig. 7.44   *Fig. 7.45*

corresponding to the amygdala. This hyperperfusion extended to the lateral parts of the left temporal lobe in a scan carried out during a series of complex partial seizures (Fig. 7.45, lower).

CASE 8

A 6-year-old boy, who had meningococcal meningitis, associated with febrile convulsions at 11 months, developed epilepsy at the age of 2 which was progressively worsening to the point where he was having several seizures per day. The seizures were typical psychomotor seizures with an aura of fear and retching. He would then go into a stare, look to the left and clench his right hand. This would be associated with hyperventilation and was followed by a period of post-ictal confusion. The seizures were entirely refractory to medical treatment.

The EEG showed seizures arising from the left side, probably the left anterior temporal region. CT scan (Fig. 7.46) showed only minimal enlargement of the left temporal horn. MRI was normal.

SPET scanning carried out interictally (Fig. 7.47, upper) demonstrated hypoperfusion of the whole of the left temporal lobe. Some reduction in flow in the left frontal lobe was also seen. The hypoperfusion of the left temporal and frontal regions became slightly more marked in a scan carried out 15 minutes post-ictally (Fig. 7.47, lower).

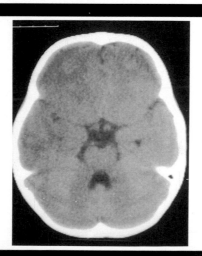

Fig. 7.46

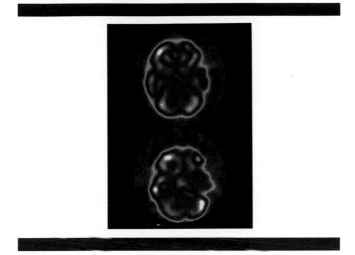

Fig. 7.17

A left temporal lobectomy was carried out and the patient is now seizure free.

CASE 9

A 20-year-old man who had a grand mal seizure at the age of 10 months. He was well until the age of 11, when he developed typical temporal lobe seizures with an epigastric aura followed by absence, then automatisms with garbled speech and post-ictal confusion and tiredness. He was tried on most anti-convulsant medications, with little effect upon his seizure frequency, which was around eight per month.

MRI scanning showed no anatomical asymmetry of the grey or white matter although there was a slight increase in the signal in the left temporal lobe on the T2 weighted scan (Fig. 7.48). EEG, ictally and interictally, was suggestive of left temporal origin seizures.

Interictal SPET (Fig. 7.49, upper) showed bilateral temporal hypoperfusion which was most prominent on the left. A repeat scan carried out $1\frac{1}{2}$ minutes after a seizure showed profound depression to flow in the left temporal lobe compared to the interictal picture.

The patient underwent left anterior temporal lobectomy and at present is seizure free.

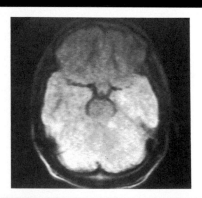

Fig. 7.48

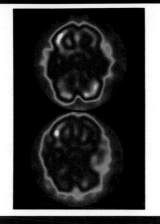

Fig. 7.49

CASE 10

A 23-year-old man who had febrile convulsions as an infant and complex partial seizures from the age of 6 with tonic clonic seizures about once a year. The seizure frequency was several per month. His complex partial seizures began with a rising feeling in the abdomen, followed by a stare, motor automatisms and confusion post-ictally. He was refractory to drug therapy. EEG recordings suggested a right-sided origin for the seizures

Fig. 7.50

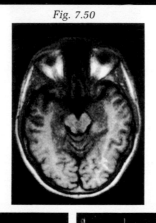

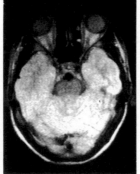

Fig. 7.51   *Fig. 7.52*

with sphenoidal electrodes suggesting a mesial temporal origin.

T1 weighted (Fig. 7.50) and T2 weighted (Figs. 7.51, 7.52) MRI scans showed no areas of abnormal signals although there was a suggestion of an abnormal amount of grey matter in the medial aspect of the left temporal lobe. Interictal SPET scanning showed an area of hyperperfusion in the lateral cortex of the right temporal lobe with possibly also a slight increase in the mesial cortex of the same side. A repeat examination carried out 1 minute postictally also demonstrated the slightly increased perfusion of the right medial cortex, but the lateral cortex then became markedly hypoperfused. This hypoperfusion extended also into the frontal region.

The patient had a right temporal lobectomy with complete relief of seizures.

CASE 11

A 21-year-old man with a history of seizures since the age of 8. The seizures were two to three per week, half being grand mal and half complex partial. He had a non-specific aura with absence and occasional automatisms. He was refractory to drug therapy and the severity of his seizures had been such that he had required residential care from time to time. EEG with foramen ovale electrode monitoring showed seizures arising from the right mesial temporal lobe. CT scanning showed a small calcified lesion in and above the right hippocampus.

MRI (Figs. 7.53, 7.54) showed a small triangular-shaped lesion in the right hippocampal region, with mixed signal on the T1 weighted sequence (Fig. 7.53) and hypointensity on the T2 weighted sequence (Fig. 7.54).

Interictally, SPET showed increased perfusion in the right mesial temporal area (Fig. 7.55, upper) which persisted in the scan carried out 1 minute post-ictally (Fig. 7.55, lower).

A right anterior temporal lobectomy was carried out and the lesion seen on CT and MRI proved to be a slow growing glioma extending into the cerebral peduncle. Post-operatively the patient's seizure frequency is much reduced.

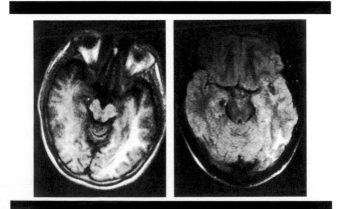

Fig. 7.53   *Fig. 7.54*

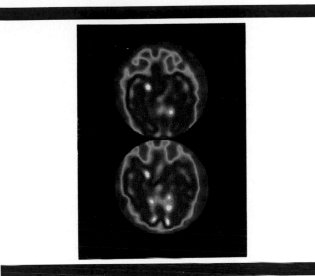

Fig. 7.55

CASE 12

A 35-year-old right-handed neurosurgeon with no symptoms or signs of disease agreed to volunteer.

In the CBF/SPET study (Fig. 7.56), transverse (top row),
coronal (middle row) and sagittal (bottom row) sections of
the brain showed a homogeneous distribution of tracer
with no perfusion deficits either at the cortical or subcortical
level. Apparent areas of relatively lower uptake/retention
of tracer can be seen in the temporal and inferior frontal
cortex. Cerebrum/cerebellum activity ratios confirm these
as variation of a normal pattern of brain perfusion.

On the top row four transverse slices at the level of (from
left to right) OM line (cerebellum), OM line + 30mm (basal
ganglia), OM line + 50mm (midventricular) and OM line +
70mm (parietal lobes) are shown. The middle row shows
four coronal slices at the level of (from left to right) frontal
lobes, basal ganglia and anterior temporal lobes, thalamus
and midparieto-temporal region, and posterior parietal and
cerebellum. The bottom row displays four sagittal slices at
the level of the right temporal lobe (1st), right basal ganglia
and thalamus (2nd), left basal ganglia and thalamus (3rd)
and left temporal lobe (4th).

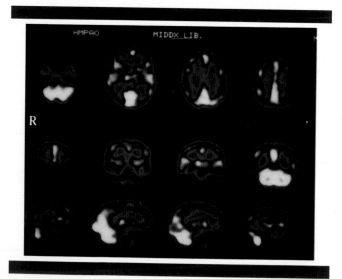

Fig. 7.56

This study shows the pattern of normal brain perfusion in a young man. Often, a semi-quantitative analysis of the distribution of the tracer is required to confirm or rule out pathology.

CASE 13

A 55-year-old right-handed male with a life-long difficulty to remember names was referred by the psychiatrist for reassurance. His psychometric testing showed scores within normal limits.

A first CT scan was reported to show a possible small lesion in the left temporal lobe. A repeat CT scan (before and after contrast) one month later demonstrated no lesions.

In the CBF/SPET study (Fig. 7.57), transverse (top row), coronal (middle row) and sagittal (bottom row) sections of the brain showed a homogeneous distribution of tracer with no perfusion deficits either at the cortical or subcortical level. The coronal slices display a uniform pattern of tracer deposition in both temporal lobes with mesial and lateral cortex surrounding the white matter and temporal horns of the lateral ventricles. Cerebrum/cerebellum activity ratios demonstrated this to be a normal brain perfusion pattern.

This study helped to reassure a forgetful, otherwise normal individual.

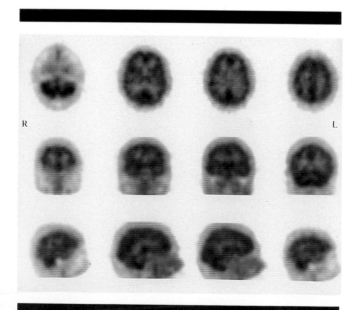

R   L

Fig. 7.57

CASE 14

An 82-year-old right-handed male agreed to undertake a HMPAO/SPET study as an age-matched normal control for his wife with a dementia of Alzheimer type (DAT). Psychometric testing scores were within normal limits for his age. A CT scan showed non-specific generalized mild cortical atrophy and mild ventricular dilatation (Fig. 7.58).

In the CBF/SPET study (Fig. 7.59), transverse (top row), coronal (middle row) and sagittal (bottom row) sections of the brain showed a homogeneous distribution of tracer with no perfusion deficits either at the cortical or subcortical level. The lateral ventricles (space between the heads of the caudate nuclei in the transverse sections) appear dilated. The temporal lobes are less well defined (particularly in the coronal slices). Cerebrum/cerebellum activity ratios are within normal limits for his age.

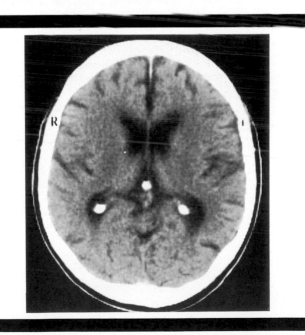

Fig. 7.58

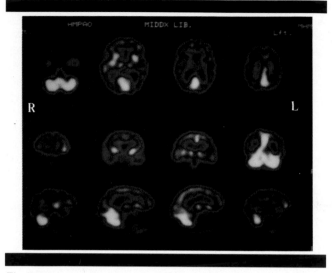

Fig. 7.59

This study clearly demonstrates the importance of quantitative methods to distinguish a normal from an abnormal perfusion pattern.

CASE 15

A 69-year-old right-handed male agreed to undertake this study as a control at the same time as his wife (DAT patient). Psychometric testing scores and CT scan were within normal limits for his age. He did not show any symptom/sign of either neuropsychiatric or other disease.

In the CBF/SPET study (Fig. 7.60), transverse (top row), coronal (middle row) and sagittal (bottom row) sections of the brain showed a homogeneous distribution of tracer with no perfusion deficits either at the cortical or subcortical level. Cerebrum/cerebellum activity ratios confirmed this to be a normal pattern of cortical and subcortical brain perfusion.

This study shows normal brain perfusion, as demonstrated by CBF/SPET.

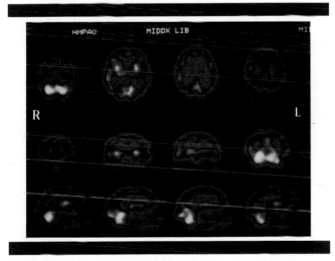

Fig. 7.60

CASE 16

A 24-year-old right-handed female with rare headache episodes and no symptom/sign of either neuropsychiatric or other disease. She volunteered for this study because of a past family history of cerebrovascular disease. At presentation for the study her blood pressure was 130/80 mmHg, heart rate 86 bpm and she was free of headache.

In the CBF/SPET study (Fig. 7.61), transverse (top row), coronal (middle row) and sagittal (bottom row) sections of the brain showed a homogeneous distribution of tracer with no perfusion deficits either at the cortical or subcortical level. The cerebrum/cerebellum activity ratios were within normal limits.

This study shows the pattern of normal brain perfusion in the cortex and subcortical structures of a young female.

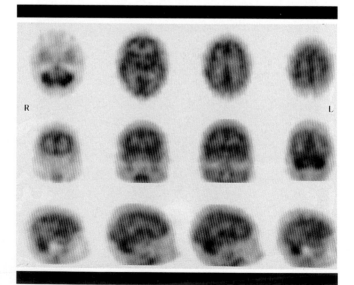

Fig. 7.61

CASE 17

A 62-year-old right-handed female with a 4-year history of apraxia/aphasia and amnesia confirmed by psychometric testing.

In the CBF/SPET study (Fig. 7.62), transverse (top row), coronal (middle row) and sagittal (bottom row) sections of the brain showed bilateral perfusion deficits in the cortex of frontal, temporal and parietal lobes. The perfusion pattern in the visual cortex, cerebellum and basal ganglia appears normal. In addition the images demonstrate worse perfusion to the left, than to the right, hemisphere. Note the advantageous display of the temporal lobe perfusion deficits in the coronal sections. In this particular case the sagittal slices demonstrate the perfusion deficits in the posterior parietal cortex as well as the transverse section.

This study shows a pattern of abnormal cortical brain perfusion characteristic of dementia of the Alzheimer type (DAT). In addition, it demonstrates bilateral impairment of the perfusion in the brain of a DAT patient with advanced disease. However, these perfusion abnormalities are asymmetric.

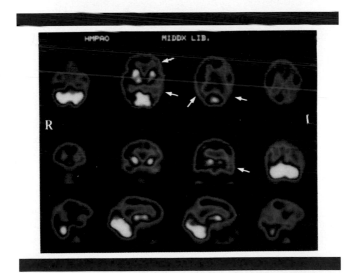

Fig. 7.62

CASE 18

A 60-year-old right-handed male with a 2-year history of DAT. The onset of the disease was 6 years before, as he started to be confused with slow deterioration of his writing and reading. Two years later the memory impairment was marked and at presentation for the study his word finding ability was severely impaired. A CT scan showed severe atrophy affecting both hemispheres with no difference between the anterior and posterior regions (Fig. 7.63). There was some ventricular dilatation and poor differentiation between grey and white matter.

In the CBF/SPET study (Fig. 7.64), transverse (top row), coronal (middle row) and sagittal (bottom row) sections of the brain showed bilateral and symmetrical perfusion deficits in the cortex of frontal, temporal and parietal lobes. This is worse in the temporal and parietal than in the frontal cortex. There is preserved perfusion to the visual

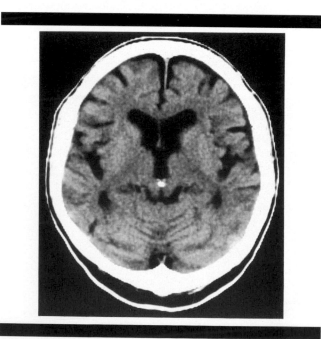

Fig. 7.63

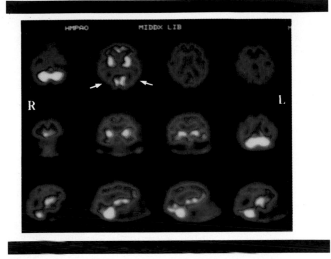

Fig. 7.64

cortex on the left hemisphere and to the basal ganglia on both sides.

This study demonstrates a characteristic bilateral and symmetrical perfusion deficiency in the brain of a DAT patient with advanced disease. There is a marked discrepancy between the cortical atrophy seen on the CT scan and the perfusion abnormalities detected with the brain perfusion study.

CASE 19

A 44-year-old right-handed male with a 1-year history of intellectual deterioration and personality changes attributed to dementia of the frontal lobe type (Pick's disease). The CT scan showed no significant abnormality, apart from a mild asymmetry of the anterior horns of the lateral ventricles (Fig. 7.65).

In the CBF/SPET study (Fig. 7.66), transverse (top row), coronal (middle row) and sagittal (bottom row) sections of the brain showed bilateral perfusion deficits confined to the frontal cortex. In addition there are mild perfusion deficits in the mesial cortex of both temporal lobes (best seen in the coronal sections) confirmed by cerebrum/cerebellum activity ratios.

The anterior horns of the lateral ventricles are slightly dilated and there is significant reduction in the perfusion

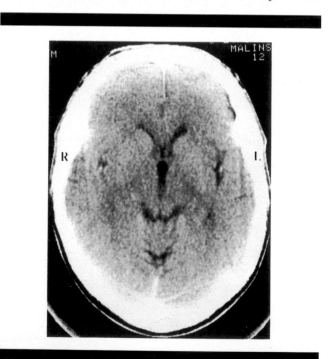

Fig. 7.65

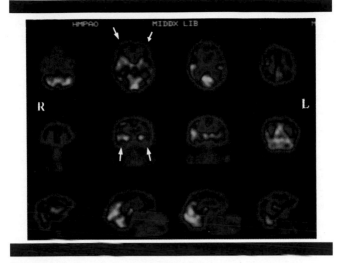

Fig. 7.60

to the heads of the caudate nuclei. The latter contrasts with the normal size of the heads of the caudate nuclei seen with the CT scan.

This study shows the pattern of abnormal cortical brain perfusion characteristic of dementia of the frontal type (Pick's disease). Marked contrast between the anatomy (CT scan) and the perfusion (SPET study) of the heads of the caudate nuclei.

CASE 20

A 68-year-old right-handed male with a 3-year history of severe impairment of his language abilities shown in reading, nominal disphasia and general difficulty in elaborating the meaning of words. Psychometric assessment showed further impairment of short-term memory. A CT scan revealed generalized cortical atrophy, particularly affecting the insular regions. The left temporal horn of the lateral ventricles was shown to be larger than the right (Fig. 7.67).

In the CBF/SPET study (Fig. 7.68), transverse (top row), coronal (middle row) and sagittal (bottom row) sections of the brain showed bilateral perfusion deficits in the temporal lobes, particularly the left. There is extension of the perfusion deficits into the posterior temporal as well as the posterior parietal cortical regions, more pronounced in the left hemisphere. It is interesting to note the relatively high tracer deposition in the skeletal muscles of the face, seen in the coronal and sagittal sections.

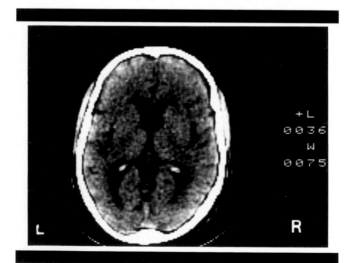

Fig. 7.67

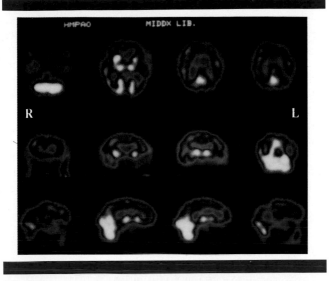

Fig. 7.68

This study shows an abnormal perfusion pattern to the temporal and posterior parietal lobes characteristic of DAT. The temporal lobe perfusion deficits are displayed best in the coronal sections.

CASE 21

A 67-year-old right-handed male with a 6-year history of cognitive impairment. He presented with apraxia, agnosia and short-term memory, scoring just 4 out of 30 on the Mini Mental State test. A CT scan showed pronounced enlargement of the lateral ventricles, particularly the anterior horns and some sulcal atrophy, more marked in the frontal cortex (Fig. 7.69).

In the CBF/SPET study (Fig. 7.70), transverse (top row), coronal (middle row) and sagittal (bottom row) sections of the brain showed bilateral and symmetrical perfusion deficits in the frontal, temporal and parietal lobes. In addition there is significant ventricular dilatation. There is no significant difference in the patterns of perfusion between the frontal and temporal/parietal lobes.

This study shows an abnormal brain perfusion pattern, bilateral and symmetrical, characteristic of DAT. There is

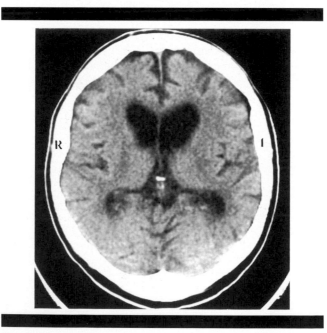

Fig. 7.69

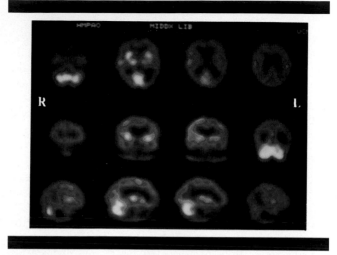

Fig. 7.70

a marked discrepancy between the cortical atrophy seen with the CT scan confined to the frontal lobes and the severe impairment of the brain perfusion in the frontal, temporal and parietal lobes.

CASE 22

A 73-year-old right-handed female with a 6-year history of DAT. She presented with pure progressive amnesia and neither dyspraxia nor dysphasia. A CT scan showed mild generalized cortical atrophy with enlargement of the anterior horns of the lateral ventricles (Fig. 7.71). Fourteen months later there was significant impairment of her intellectual performance. The amnesia was more severe and there was apraxia and agnosia.

The first study demonstrated the mild ventricular enlargement and a single well defined perfusion abnormality confined to the right temporal lobe (coronal section). However, there is a less marked perfusion deficit in the mesial cortex of the left temporal lobe (Fig. 7.72, upper). This was confirmed by the cerebrum/cerebellum activity ratios.

The repeat study (14 months later) revealed further impairment of the perfusion to both temporal lobes and frontal lobes, with less marked deficient perfusion to the

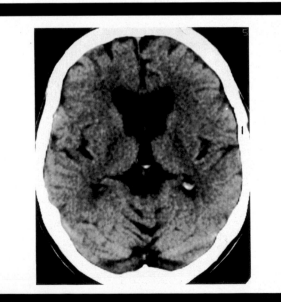

Fig. 7.71

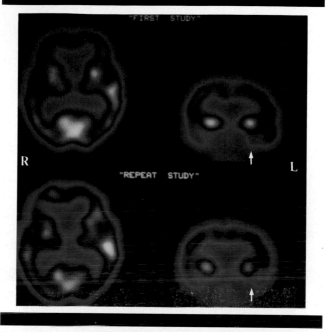

Fig. 7.72

right parietal cortex (Fig. 7.72, lower). Cerebrum/cerebellum activity ratios confirmed these further abnormalities of perfusion in the areas described. The coronal sections display the temporal lobe deficits and the transverse slices show the frontal cortex abnormalities.

These studies reveal a hint of the natural progression of DAT, starting in the temporal lobes and progressing later to the parietal and frontal cortex.

CASE 23

A 66-year-old right-handed male with a long history of chronic alcoholism and more recent (1 year) memory loss. An EEG showed generalized increase in theta only. A CT scan revealed generalized cortical atrophy and no focal areas of mass attenuation.

In the CBF/SPET study (Fig. 7.73), transverse (top row), coronal (middle row) and sagittal (bottom row) sections of the brain showed bilateral perfusion deficits sparing the cerebellum and visual cortex. The lateral ventricles appeared enlarged. The basal ganglia and brain stem showed a relatively preserved perfusion pattern.

Frontal, parietal and temporal lobes are severely affected by disease.

This study shows an abnormal perfusion pattern compatible with dementia of Alzheimer type, rather than alcohol-induced dementia.

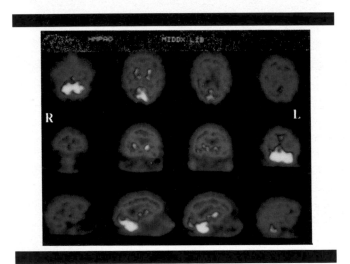

Fig. 7.73

CASE 24

A 66-year-old right-handed female was admitted for the investigation of peripheral vascular disease. On clinical examination she was found to have bilateral carotid bruits and a pan-arteriogram showed stenosis of the right common iliac artery, a plaque at the origin of the left common iliac artery and marked stenosis of both internal carotid arteries at the bifurcartion and beyond. During admission she had an episode of loss of vision on the right side and was referred for a brain perfusion study. The carotid angiogram (DSA) (Fig. 7.74) shows the internal carotid stenosis, bilaterally.

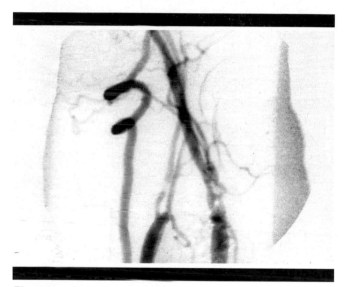

Fig. 7.74

The CBF/SPET study (Fig. 7.75) demonstrated a single small perfusion deficit in the right occipital cortex (arrow), extending into the posterior parietal cortex. No crossed cerebellar diaschisis is noticed. The top row (from left to right) shows four transverse slices at the level of orbito-meatal (OM) line (cerebellum), OM line + 30mm (basal ganglia), OM line + 50 mm (midventricular section) and OM line + 60mm. The bottom row displays, from the left to the right, coronal slices at the level of the frontal lobe (1st), basal ganglia (2nd), midtemporo-parietal region and thalamus (3rd) and posterior parietal and cerebellum (4th).

This study indicates that when SPET studies are carried out early after CVD, pathology can be demonstrated which remains silent on CT or/and MRI.

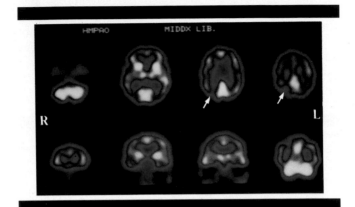

Fig. 7.75

CASE 25

A 59-year-old right-handed retired male teacher was admitted with a 9-month history of left leg hemiparesis. This was of gradual onset and had become stable shortly afterwards (2 months). There was a past history (13 years before) of cerebrovascular disease with an episode of dysphasia, right homonymous hemianopia, dysgraphia and dyslexia from which he did not recover.

A CT brain scan showed a mature infarct in the left parietal and occipital lobes, and a lacuna in the left thalamus (Fig. 7.76). Minor cortical atrophy was apparent with no focal abnormalities seen in the right hemisphere.

The CBF/SPET study demonstrated a large perfusion abnormality in the left parietal and occipital lobes, in keeping with the established cerebral infarct seen in the CT scan. In addition there was an asymmetry of the thalamic perfusion (L<R), and crossed cerebellar diaschisis was demonstrated (Fig. 7.77).

The relatively lower perfusion of the right high parietal lobe explains the clinical presentation.

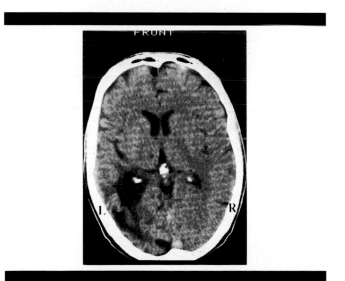

Fig. 7.76

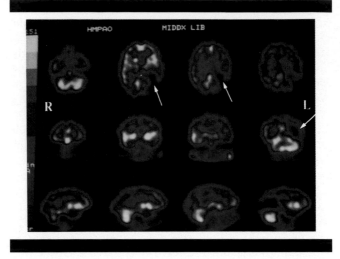

Fig. 7.77

This study shows that CT scan of the brain will document anatomical abnormalities. CBF/SPET studies will document the dynamic nature of the perfusion insult and its evolution.

CASE 26

A 64-year-old female was admitted for the investigation of increasing angina over the past 6 years despite intensive medical treatment. Coronary angiogram demonstrated a severe 80% stenosis in the proximal anterior descending artery (LAD), a very severe stenosis (>90%) in the main stem of the left circumflex (LCx) and diffuse irregularities of a dominant right coronary artery (RCA). She underwent coronary artery bypass graft (CABG) to the LAD and LCx arteries. The day after surgery she developed paresis of the right arm and leg with no abnormality of facial muscles, speech or comprehension. A few hours later she recovered the right hand power. No change in the right leg paresis was noticed.

A CT scan revealed a cerebral infarction in the left high parietal cortex, close to the interhemispheric groove (Fig. 7.78).

The CBF/SPET study demonstrated a single small perfusion deficit in the left high parietal cortex (arrow), close to the midline, seen on the transverse (Fig. 7.79A)

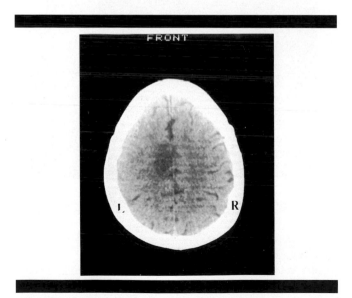

Fig. 7.78

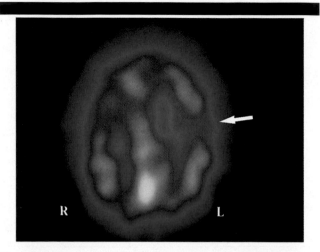

Fig. 7.79A

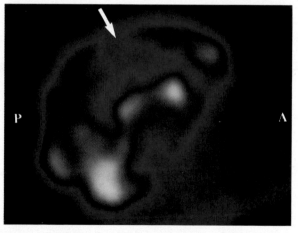

Fig. 7.79B

and sagittal (Fig. 7.79B) slices, with no other abnormalities detected.

Cerebral vascular events are a frequent unwanted outcome from coronary artery surgery. Brain perfusion SPET studies may help to choose the candidates for surgery as well as to follow-up their response to treatment.

CASE 27

A 64-year-old right-handed female was admitted via casualty with left-sided weakness of face and arm. On examination there was left-sided sensory and visual inattention. Six days later she recovered considerably and only a mild left-arm weakness was noticeable. A CT scan performed 8 days on admission revealed a large inferior frontal low density lesion with minor mass effect relative to its size and with only minimal peripheral enhancement (Fig. 7.80). A DSA on the following day demonstrated complete obstruction of the origin of the right internal carotid artery (Fig. 7.81). There was extensive colateral intracraneal flow and a large atheromatous plaque at the origin of the left internal carotid artery. She was referred for a CBF/SPET study in order to evaluate the brain perfusion pattern in both hemispheres before carotid surgery was planned.

The CBF/SPET study was carried out on day 10 of admission. It showed reduced perfusion in the right frontal and parietal cortex with increased tracer distribution in the surrounding cortical brain structures (watershed zone) (Fig. 7.82, upper). A repeat study (without any further tracer injection) was undertaken in the same day, 5 hours after the tracer administration. It revealed a partial wash-

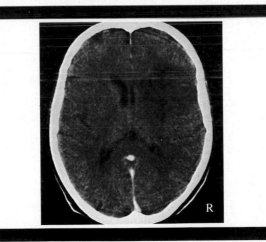

Fig. 7.80

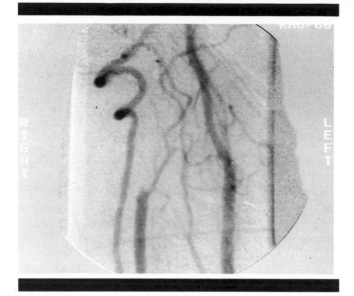

Fig. 7.81

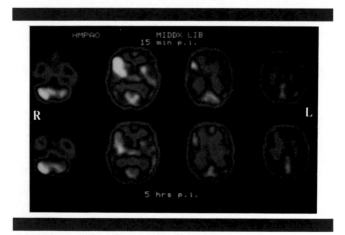

Fig. 7.82

out from the watershed area with still increased distribution (retention) of tracer (Fig. 7.82, lower). This was probably dependent on the presence of viable cerebral tissue

which in conjunction with the improvement in this patient's clinical condition indicated good prognosis.

Repeat CBF/SPET studies in cases of ischaemic cerebral lesions may allow for the assessment of viable cerebral tissue and hence contribute to a prognostic score.

CASE 28

An 81-year-old right-handed male was referred with drowsiness, left hemiplegia, inattention in the left arm and hand reflexes, one year after an acute right fronto-parietal cerebral cortex infarction. There were no speech changes. A CT scan performed at time of onset of disease had shown an ill-defined area of low density in the right fronto-parietal region compatible with a cerebral infarction (Fig. 7.83). The CBF/SPET study was requested to assess progression of disease due to communication difficulties (patient speaks a difficult local foreign dialect).

The CBF/SPET study (Fig. 7.84) showed areas of severely reduced cortical perfusion in the right hemisphere in the frontal and parietal lobes. Transverse (top row), coronal (middle row) and sagittal (bottom row) sections clearly demonstrated this perfusion abnormality, particularly affecting the right frontal lobe. In addition, it revealed the viable tissue surrounding this well established lesion. No significant crossed cerebellar diaschisis was observed.

It is interesting to notice that planar views (Fig. 7.85) of

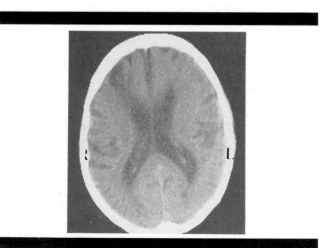

Fig. 7.83

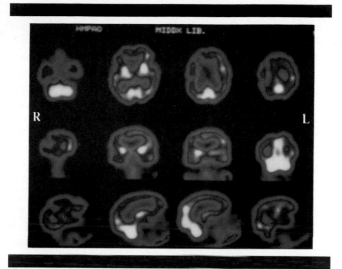

Fig. 7.84

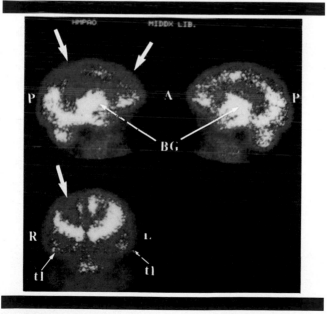

Fig. 7.85

the distribution of the tracer in the brain distinctly identified the different cortical areas (particularly the temporal lobes [tl] and basal ganglia [BG]) as well as the perfusion abnormality in the right hemisphere (arrow). This was mainly due to the significant cortical atrophy and lateral ventricles (anterior, posterior and temporal horns) dilatation.

This study highlights the contribution of SPET to the documentation of altered physiology (perfusion) in the brain. Extension abnormalities on SPET occur in the presence of mild or moderate changes in the CT study.

CASE 29

A 54-year-old right-handed female was admitted via casualty with a flaccid right-sided hemiplegia 3 days after the onset of occipital headache, vomit, aphasia and right-sided severe hemiplegia. A CT scan performed within less than 12 hours of onset was unremarkable (Fig. 7.86). Another CT scan on admission demonstrated an extensive low density area involving the basal ganglia, internal capsule and lateral frontal lobe on the left side. The left lateral ventricle appeared compressed. A DSA performed on day 24 of onset depicted a severe stricture of the left internal carotid associated with a small distal vessel and very delayed flow (Fig. 7.87).

The CBF/SPET study on day 13 of onset demonstrated the area of cerebral infarction with increased tracer deposition in the watershed area ('luxury perfusion') (Fig. 7.88, upper). There was crossed cerebellar diaschisis and the basal ganglia were seen with good perfusion pattern. On day 40 of onset, with no significant change in the neurological clinical condition, the SPET study was

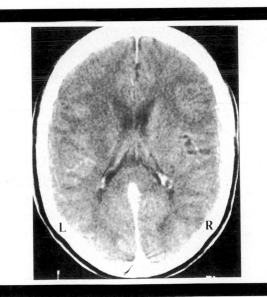

Fig. 7.86

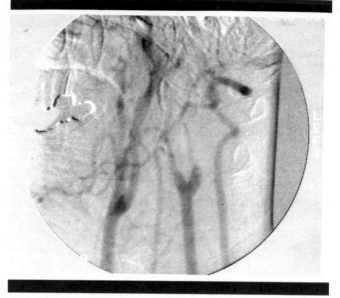

Fig. 7.87

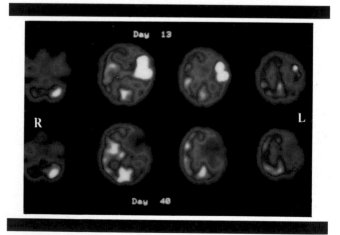

Fig. 7.88

repeated to assess progression of disease. It demonstrated a large area of severely deficient perfusion in the left fronto-parietal and deep temporal lobes, involving the ipsilateral basal ganglia and sparing the thalamus (Fig. 7.88, lower). Crossed cerebellar diaschisis was still present.

There is some debate regarding the significance of 'luxury perfusion'. Unfortunately in this case it was not possible to repeat the first CBF/SPET later in the day to assess the presence or absence of washout.

CASE 30

A 53-year-old right-handed male with left hemiplegia of sudden onset due to a right fronto-parietal metastasis from a renal cell carcinoma. A CT scan was performed the same day of the SPET study and demonstrated the lesion surrounded by a large area of oedema (Fig. 7.89A,B).

In the CBF/SPET study (Fig. 7.90), transverse (top row), coronal (middle row) and sagittal (bottom row) sections of

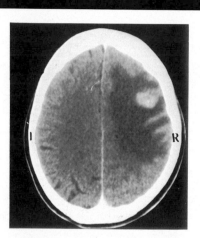

Fig. 7.89A

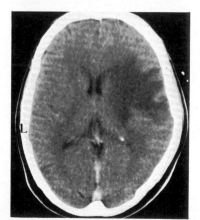

Fig. 7.89B

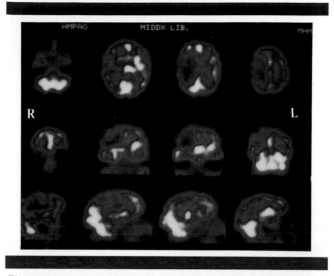

Fig. 7.90

the brain showed severe reduction in the perfusion to the right hemisphere. There was crossed cerebellar diaschisis. Although the metastasis itself was not demonstrated, the perfusion abnormality was in keeping with the clinical neurological findings. The perfusion abnormality matched the extent of oedema seen with the CT scan. However, it appeared even larger than in the CT scan.

CBF/SPET studies of brain perfusion can provide evidence of the extent of altered physiology in keeping with neurological symptoms and signs. Brain perfusion studies demonstrate the effect of neoplasia, usually seen as a large area of impaired perfusion/flow surrounding the primary or secondary tumour.

CASE 31

A 40-year-old male with a left temporal lobe epileptic focus on surface EEG and a normal CT brain scan was referred for a CBF/SPET study.

The CBF/SPET study clearly demonstrated a significant reduction in the perfusion to the left temporal, seen in the transverse and coronal slices (Fig. 7.91). Reorientation of the transverse slices (Fig. 7.92) permitted the temporal cortex to be seen with some perfusion, surrounding an area of absent tracer deposition (arrow). MRI performed *a posteriori* depicted a small glioma in the left temporal lobe.

Long axis display sections of the temporal lobes is optimal for the localization and lateralization of perfusion abnormalities in this area of the brain.

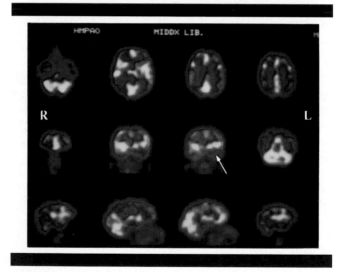

Fig. 7.91

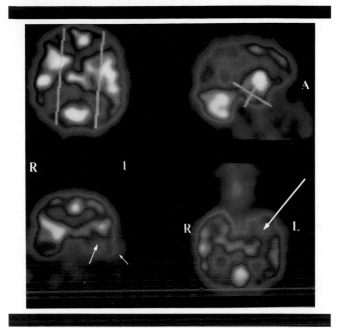

Fig. 7.92

CASE 32

A 31-year-old male diver with a history of mild cerebral symptoms after an emergency ascent in 1985. Lung function studies showed areas of poor compliance. He made a full clinical recovery and was referred for a CBF/SPET study to assess possible risk of further diving.

In the CBF/SPET study (Fig. 7.93), transverse (top row) and coronal (bottom row) sections of the brain showed areas of severe deficit in the perfusion of both frontal, parietal (more on the left hemisphere) and temporal lobes. The lateral ventricles were dilated and there was lower tracer deposition in the head of caudate nuclei, as well as the brain stem.

Severe cortical brain damage has been found in divers. CBF/SPET studies demonstrate utility in the assessment of populations at special risk (divers, pilots, etc.). In this particular case there is a striking discrepancy between clinical status and the degree of perfusion impairment. The patient was advised to stop further diving.

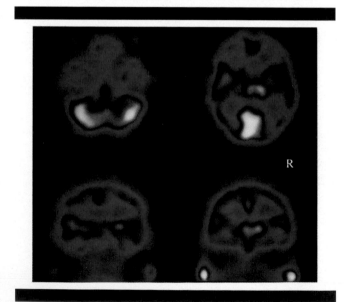

Fig. 7.93

CASE 33

A 13-year-old female with Gilles de la Tourette syndrome and attention disorder deficit in addition to coprolalia, copropraxia and echophenomena was referred for a CBF/ SPET study.

In the CBF/SPET study (Fig. 7.94), transverse (top row) and coronal (bottom row) sections of the brain showed slightly enlarged ventricles for her age. In addition, there was reduction in the perfusion to the cortex of the frontal, parietal and temporal lobes. Asymmetry of the tracer uptake in the head of the caudate nuclei (Fig. 7.94, lower left) was observed. This has been confirmed by quantification using the cerebellum for normalization.

Abnormal brain perfusion in patients with Gilles de la Tourette syndrome can be identified. Interestingly these perfusion changes seem to involve more frequently the basal ganglia. There are large variations in the extent of cortical involvement and CBF impairment in these patients.

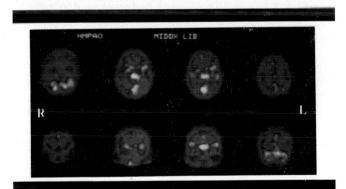

Fig. 7.94

CASE 34

An 11-year-old male with Gilles de la Tourette syndrome with attention deficit disorder and hyperactivity (ADDH), as well as vocal tics (coprolalia, copropraxia and echophenomena), but no family history, was referred for a CBF/ SPET study.

In the CBF/SPET study (Fig. 7.95), transverse (top row), coronal (middle row) and sagittal (bottom row) sections of the brain showed slightly enlarged ventricles for his age. In addition, there was reduction in the perfusion to the mesial cortex of the temporal lobes, to the left parietal lobe and asymmetry of the tracer uptake in the head of the caudate nuclei (Fig. 7.95, lower left).

Abnormal brain perfusion in patients with Gilles de la Tourette syndrome can be identified. Interestingly, these perfusion changes seem to involve more frequently the basal ganglia.

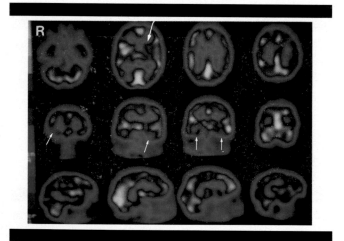

Fig. 7.95

Index

Index